Reduce Your Breast Cancer Risks

Reduce Your Breast Cancer Risks

Basic Facts Plus Four Simple Changes That Work

Joyce C. Smolkin, M.A., M.S.

Writer's Showcase
San Jose New York Lincoln Shanghai

Reduce Your Breast Cancer Risks
Basic Facts Plus Four Simple Changes That Work

Writer's Showcase
an imprint of iUniverse.com, Inc.

For information address:
iUniverse.com, Inc.
5220 S 16th, Ste. 200
Lincoln, NE 68512
www.iuniverse.com

The purpose of this book is to educate and provide information in the areas covered. The information contained herein is based on the author's research and is not intended to be a substitute or alternative for appropriate medical advice or treatment. The reader should consult with a physician or health care provider prior to utilizing any course of action or treatment mentioned in this book.

It should be noted that as a result of continuing research and technology, new findings may change or invalidate some of the data presented.

The author and publisher hereby disclaim any responsibility or liability, personal or otherwise, that is incurred from the use or application of this book.

ISBN: 0-595-15831-5

Printed in the United States of America

Dedication

To my husband, Stanley, without whose love and continuing support this book would not have been written

To my sons, Mark and Matthew, and daughter-in-law Robyn for the joy they bring to my life

To my mother, Lillian, who as a forerunner in stressing the importance of proper diet and regular exercise helped me lead the life I now promote

To my father, Melvin, who loved to write, and inspired me to follow my dreams

To my in-laws, Rita and Morris, who have always treated me like a daughter

And to all the women I've met during my breast cancer journey that have changed my life for the better, and provided me with the impetus for writing this book

Epigraph

We wholly conquer only what we assimilate.

Gide

Contents

Foreword

Breast cancer is the most frequently diagnosed cancer in women in the United States, accounting for 182,800 new cases and 40,800 deaths in 2000. The risk of developing breast cancer increases with age and it is estimated that in a woman's lifetime, approximately 1 in 8 will develop breast cancer. With increasing medical knowledge and awareness, breast cancer can be diagnosed and treated at an earlier stage improving overall prognosis. A recent very large research trial demonstrated that women who took a medication called Tamoxifen rather than a placebo reduced their risk of breast cancer. Tamoxifen had side effects that were serious enough to limit the universal use of this drug at this time, but for high-risk women this is a proven treatment. Smoking cessation, weight control, stress management, physical activity and reducing alcohol intake are other ways that have been suggested to be beneficial in reducing the risk of breast cancer.

The American Cancer Society recommends three methods for early detection of breast cancer: physical examination by a physician, mammography, and breast self-examination. Their guidelines include annual mammography and physical exam for women greater than 40 years old, and monthly breast self-exam for all greater than 20 years old. Because 15 percent of all breast cancers are not found on routine mammograms, it is very important for all women to perform monthly breast self-examination.

The author discusses ways to reduce the risk for breast cancer and offers tips for maintaining good health. If the readers follow the recommendations in this book they would not only reduce their risk for breast cancer, but also for other cancers as well as heart disease and diabetes. It is especially educational and informative about nutritional habits and helpful cooking hints for a healthier diet as well as exercise and stress management.

Good diet, reduced stress, increased physical activity, and the cessation of smoking are important lifestyle changes that cannot be overemphasized in our modern fast-paced society.

M. Margaret Kemeny, M.D., F.A.C.S
Chief, Division of Surgical Oncology
University Hospital and Health Sciences Center
Stony Brook, New York

Acknowledgements

I want to thank the following individuals for their support, suggestions, and assistance—

Mark Smolkin for his editing suggestions

Anna Tullis for her unbridled encouragement that kept me going

Leslie Pierno, Fran Oprosko, and Kathleen Emmett for their valid opinions

Ralph Horowitz for much needed computer assistance

Introduction

Life is an exciting adventure filled with many unknowns including those unforeseen and unsolicited assaults to our health. When confronted by these challenges we must be willing to deal with them head-on, even when they are frightening and life threatening.

In August 1995 I discovered a lump in my breast. After a getting a mammogram and a sonogram, I went with the films in hand to a surgeon who did a needle biopsy, and confirmed my worst fears—I had breast cancer. Since I was the first female in my family to receive this diagnosis, the unanticipated results threw me for a loop. After allowing the news to sink in, I proceeded to learn more about the protocol that would best serve my needs. Finally, I underwent treatment—lumpectomy, chemotherapy, and radiation—a standard combination for Stage 1 breast cancer when estrogen and progesterone negative tumor receptors are present.

While it was not an experience anyone can really prepare for, I'm convinced that my healthy lifestyle—I'm a longtime vegetarian who exercises regularly and maintains a proper weight—worked to my advantage. Although both environmental and personal risk factors may have contributed to the growth of my cancer, I attribute the diagnosis in part to my struggle with excess stress during the preceding five years—returning to school to complete undergraduate and graduate degrees, working, managing a household, and caring long-distance for aged parents. I truly believe this combination played a role in the breakdown of my immune system, allowing the hidden cancer cells to proliferate.

It didn't take me long to realize that being diagnosed with breast cancer was not a fait accompli but rather a time to re-evaluate my life. I envisioned myself perched at the edge of a precipice where I could either tumble down or fight to regain my balance and purposefully move forward in a more rewarding direction—without hesitation the latter was my action of choice. Already aware of the fact that the combination of a regular breast health program, a nutritionally sound diet, and daily exercise were all essential components of a healthy lifestyle, I acknowledged that stress reduction needed to be part of the package.

Both during and after treatment I spoke to dozens of women, some of whom were diagnosed with breast cancer, and others not touched by the disease. Many of the women were seeking information and support to assist them in making health-promoting changes to reduce their risk of developing breast cancer. This prompted me to write a program offering women the assistance they were looking for. After presenting the program in various locales, I realized that the potential audience was much larger than the one I was reaching. The next logical step was to communicate the information in book form.

The goal of *Reduce Your Breast Cancer Risks: Basic Facts, Plus Four Simple Changes That Work* is to simplify the data women have received about breast cancer, and to help them acquire and maintain a healthy lifestyle, even if they haven't arrived at a "precipice" in their own lives. Once having implemented the requisite changes the resource section will aid in continuing the process.

As an optimist, I include myself in the group of dreamers who anticipate the day when breast cancer will be eradicated, and added to the list of diseases like polio and smallpox, which for the most part no longer exist. To make this dream a reality we must all work together—the Federal Government funding the research; researchers working toward their goal of finding a cure; health care providers undertaking management of the disease; and women like you and I who in large part can contribute toward the state of our own health by improving our lifestyle, reducing our risks, and ultimately increasing our opportunity for living a long and healthy life.

Chapter 1
Understanding the Risks

As women, we are constantly reminded of our risk for developing breast cancer. Between a bombardment of daily media offerings on the latest treatment and prevention studies suggesting the possibility of a future free of this dreaded disease, to both favorable and some not so favorable statistics, it's virtually impossible for the average person to sort out all the data. Instead of helping, this flood of information frightens many women, and may ultimately keep them from following up on prescribed health benefiting programs.

On a positive note, results from recently completed studies either indicate several drugs may have a preventive effect, or suggest the answer for some women lies in gene manipulation, still in the testing stages. The goal of this chapter is to clarify some of the more newsworthy studies and protocols, and provide a general, yet understandable, overview of possible breast cancer risks.

WHAT THE DATA IS TELLING US

Breast cancer is the leading form of cancer diagnosed in women and the second leading cause of cancer death in women after lung cancer. Examination of risk variation within the United States population finds the incidence of breast cancer lowest for women of Asian and Hispanic decent, and highest for Caucasian women overall, one exception being African-American women under the age of 50 who have the highest rates.[1][2] Statistically breast cancer incidence increased, on average, one percent a year between 1940 and 1982, and 4 percent a year from 1982 to 1987.[3] From 1990 to 1994 the rates stabilized at approximately 110 per 100,000 for the general population[4] (where it remains today), and 101.5 per 100,000 for African-American women.[5] A large portion of this leveling off is attributable to better diagnostic tools, and increasing numbers of women getting mammograms.

An estimated 192,200 women will be diagnosed with breast cancer in the year 2001, or approximately 30 percent of all newly diagnosed cancer cases for all sites. [6] Of those women diagnosed, almost 40 percent will require more invasive treatment because cancer cells have moved from the breast to the lymph nodes and other parts of the body. This data suggests we still have a long way to go to convince women of the importance of participating in an early detection protocol, and maintaining a healthy lifestyle.

We still don't fully understand why the breast cancer rates are so high, especially for older women. The reasons most frequently suggested include: 1) more women living well into their postmenopausal years; 2) increasing numbers of women going for mammograms and being diagnosed with breast cancer (although at an earlier stage than if they had postponed their mammogram); 3) modern reproductive patterns of delayed first birth and fewer children; and 4) environmental factors which increase exposure to chemicals in our food, air and water.

But there's good news too. The overall death rates from breast cancer in the United States decreased by 6.3 percent between 1991 and 1995— women under age 65 had a reduction of 9.3 percent, and Caucasian women 6.6 percent. Lesser reductions of 1.6 percent were achieved overall for African-Americans, with 2.8 percent for those women age 65 and older. Early detection, where a tumor is likely to be found at a more treatable stage, and the increased use of adjuvant (additional) therapy may account for a substantial portion of this decrease.[7]

Researchers continue to seek an answer to the question of why African-American women have higher death rates. It's believed that multiple factors contribute to their mortality rates including: 1) development of an aggressive, less treatable form of breast cancer; 2) diagnosis after the disease has already metastasized (spread to other parts of the body); 3) greater occurrence of poorly differentiated (irregular cells) tumors; 4) multiple disease contributing factors, e.g. high blood pressure, obesity and diabetes; and (5) socioeconomic conditions.[8]

We still have a long way to go in reducing the barriers to good health care for all women of color. The specific needs of these women must be addressed to increase their likelihood of using essential health-promoting strategies, including eating a nutritionally balanced diet, attaining and maintaining an appropriate weight, participating in some form of regular exercise, and getting yearly mammograms beginning at age 40. In the case of African-American women, having a baseline mammogram at age 35 or earlier is a good idea, especially when there is a family history of the disease. With these changes, and others, subsequent data are bound to denote a decline in mortality.

RISK FACTORS

When examining the risks, focus is typically centered on the fact that every woman has a 1 in 8 chance of developing breast cancer. The truth is the 1 in 8 figure relates to a woman's risk over *an entire lifetime*. This recurring message feeds into the fear many women have of receiving a positive diagnosis. Consequently, they resist going for a yearly mammogram, avoid doing breast self-examination, and most frightening of all don't schedule an appointment with their health care provider when changes in the breast become evident.

Initial scrutiny of the various risk factors can be quite disconcerting. But remember, while certain risks may appear to apply in individual situations, there is no way of knowing whether they actually do. Truthfully, every woman has some risk for developing breast cancer—the most obvious one is simply being a female.

Lifetime Risk of Developing Breast Cancer

By age 30. . . 1 out of 2,212
By age 40. . . 1 out of 235
By age 50. . . 1 out of 54
By age 60. . . 1 out of 23
By age 70. . . 1 out of 14
By age 80. . . 1 out of 10
Ever. . . . . . . 1 out of 8

Source: NCI

Young women in their 20s and 30s are less likely to be diagnosed with breast cancer. Yet, in spite of a low occurrence rate, once diagnosed, their prognosis is generally poorer than it is for older, postmenopausal women because higher levels of estrogen in pre-menopausal women increase the likelihood the tumors will be fast growing. [9] It's likely that for women in this age group unless a lump is found through breast self-examination, because of noticeable changes in the breast tissue, or simply by chance a cancer may not be detected in the early stages. Unfortunately, young women, and even their health care providers, often brush aside the emergence of obvious breast changes—taking a wait-and-see attitude. *Remember—every woman is at risk regardless of age.* Whenever a change is noted, women must pursue answers they are comfortable with, even if it means going for a second or third opinion.

Between ages 40 to 50 the risk for developing breast cancer increases more than four-fold. This rise in incidence is followed by a less rapid climb through the subsequent decades—fueling the emphasis presently being placed on having a first mammogram at age 40 to increase a woman's chances of an early diagnosis.

Whether a woman between the ages of 40 and 49 has a mammogram yearly or semi-annually is between her and her doctor. But keep in mind since breast tissue is typically denser for women in this age group, a yearly mammogram increases the likelihood a lump will be detected. After age 50 the annual mammogram is a must.

The task of estimating personal risk has been made easier with the use of the computerized Breast Cancer Risk Assessment tool (BCRA), developed by the National Cancer Institute (NCI). The BCRA aids a woman, with her doctor's help, in assessing the odds of developing breast cancer both within the next five years and over a lifetime. A rough estimate of a woman's risk is determined by calculating several key factors: present age; age at onset of menstruation; age at which she first gave birth; the number of breast cancer incidents diagnosed in her mother and sisters; the number of breast biopsies she has undergone and their results; and race.

The program does have assessment limitations, which can result in underestimation for high-risk women—it fails to take into account the age of onset of breast cancer among relatives diagnosed with breast cancer (if they were diagnosed after menopause her risk is not affected), or the history of breast cancer in her father's family (both the mother's and father's family histories assist in uncovering a woman's genetic history).

Risk Factors for Breast Cancer in Women			
Factor	High Risk	Low Risk	Relative Risk*
Age	Old	Young	>4.0
Country of birth	North American Northern Europe	Asia Africa	2.0 – 4.0
Socioeconomic status	Upper	Lower	2.0 – 4.0
Marital status	Never Married	Ever married	1.1 – 1.9
Place of residence	Urban	Rural	1.1 – 1.9
Race	White	Black	1.1 – 1.9
Age at first pregnancy	Older than 30	Younger than 20	2.0 – 4.0
No breast feeding	Yes	No	2.0 – 4.0
Oophorectomy (removal of ovaries)	No	Yes	2.0 – 4.0
Body build, postmenopausal	Obese	Thin	2.0 – 4.0
Pesticide exposure	Yes	No	2.0 – 4.0
Age at menarche	Early	Late	1.1 – 1.9
Family history of premenopausal bilateral breast cancer	Yes	No	> 4.0
History of cancer in one breast	Yes	No	> 4.0
History of fibrocystic disease (proliferative)	Yes	No	2.0 – 4.0
First-degree relative with breast cancer	Yes	No	2.0 – 4.0
History of primary cancer in ovary or endometrium	Yes	No	2.0 – 4.0
Radiation to chest	Large doses	Minimal exposure	2.0 – 4.0

Eliott, M. Special Report. Search for a Killer: Focus shifts from fat to hormones. *Science*, 1993: 259, 616-618 * Relative risk ratio suggests the disease rate among population exposed to the disease and unexposed population. For example, relative risk of 4 implies old age causes a 4 times greater risk of getting breast

Hormonal Risks

A woman's estrogen levels typically remain steady into her 40s. Perimenopause, indicative of approaching menopause, frequently causes these levels to fluctuate, sometimes erratically. Menstrual cycle irregularity can result in a variety of changes, e.g. multiple periods each month, or skipped or lengthy periods, all of which are capable of making a woman's life miserable. When problems occur, a physician may suggest beginning estrogen replacement therapy (ERT) to bring hormone levels into balance, and to allow a woman to reclaim a more normal life.

At some point, usually in her early 50s—it can vary by as much as ten years or more—a woman enters menopause, which is evidenced by a decline in estrogen levels.

> **Menopause:** *To varying degrees, women may experience symptoms related to reduced estrogen, including: hot flashes; vaginal dryness; anxiety; depression; and memory impairment.*

Low estrogen level means the woman's risk for heart disease, stroke, and Type I osteoporosis—brought about by an accelerated loss of minerals from her bones—can influence the decision to begin ERT. Unfortunately, continuing to provide a steady supply of estrogen beyond termination of the body's own resources can also increase the likelihood of, *but by no means guarantees*, a diagnosis of breast cancer. Consequently, it becomes a toss-up between "do I", or "don't I". Natural estrogens are also available and worth investigating, as are approaches other than hormone therapy, such as herbal supplements (before taking any combination of herbs check with a trained professional, whether it be your regular physician, a Chinese herbalist, or a complementary health care provider). A woman's physiological needs and the advisability of beginning ERT are derived from evaluating multiple risk factors, and should be assessed by the woman, together with her physician, when attempting to estimate her likelihood of developing breast cancer. Keep in mind, there's uncertainty about just how much of a role each risk factor actually plays and which symbiotic relationships are the most detrimental.

Early Menstruation: Menstruation beginning at age 12 or younger increases a woman's risk for breast cancer. In western countries the average age of menarche is presently 12-1/2 years, down from the historical average of 16 to 17 years of age. Today, in the United States and other developed countries, it's not uncommon for girls as young as 8 or 9 years of age to begin experiencing the hormonal changes that are precursors to menstruation. The prevalence of hormonal changes in these young girls is believed due, in part, to our society's standard way of eating—the high fat, low fiber diet. In countries where high fiber foods are eaten on a regular basis the start of menstruation is typically delayed. [10]

Late Menopause: Menstruating for forty years or more, well into their 50s, increases women's risk. There's little doubt that excessive amounts of estrogen over a long period of time has a negative effect.[11] But unless they resort to drugs or surgery women are left playing a waiting game until menopause arrives.

Nulliparity: Continuous exposure to estrogen can be a factor in abnormal cell growth in both the reproductive organs and breast tissue for women who have never given birth, or are past the age where it's likely to occur. Many women add to this estrogen overload by taking birth control pills.

Late First Pregnancy: Today, many women choose to wait until their careers are on track, or until they're financially secure enough to manage the expense of raising a child. It's not uncommon for women in their 30s, 40s, and even 50s to give birth to their first child. Delaying motherhood until after age 30 predisposes these women to an increased risk.

Age: The likelihood of a breast cancer diagnosis increases after age 50, especially if the women are postmenopausal—with over 77 percent of all diagnoses occurring beyond this point. In spite of this increased risk, many older women postpone being examined by their health care provider and have never gone for a mammogram either because of fear of diagnosis, or the belief that they personally have nothing to worry about. The reasons they most often give are likely to include, "I've lived this long without getting breast cancer, so I'll take my chances", or "no one in my family has ever had breast cancer." Unfortunately, by the time they're finally diagnosed the disease may have advanced to the point where a poor prognosis is almost guaranteed. The good news is that even when post-menopausal and diagnosed with a tumor that is both less aggressive and in an early stage, a woman is more likely to die of old age, or from a disease other than breast cancer.

Prior breast biopsies: The majority of breast biopsies find benign breast lumps. However, one particular benign growth, *atypical hyperplasia* (increased breast cell growth), which is found in approximately 3 percent of breast biopsies, is considered to increase a woman's risk of breast cancer.

Personal history of breast cancer: A woman with a prior history of breast cancer has an increased risk of developing a new cancer in the other breast. This is not the same as a recurrence of the first cancer.

Familial Risks

A family history of breast cancer on either her mother's or father's side increases a woman's risk. The greatest familial risk occurs when a mother, sister or daughter (first-degree relative) has been diagnosed with breast cancer prior to menopause. Learning of a family member's breast cancer diagnosis is especially distressing. But if it's not a first-degree relative a woman's risk is not increased—it is the same 12-1/2 percent lifetime risk as women with no family history of the disease, particularly if the relative's initial diagnosis occurred after menopause.

Genetic Risks

Genetic researchers are seeking to develop specific therapies that reduce cell replication by tapping into the biology of cancer cells. Two genes, *BRCA1* and *BRCA2*, have already been identified as the culprits involved in increasing the risk of breast, ovarian, and prostate cancer, primarily for members of the Ashkenazi (Eastern European) Jewish community.

According to the principal investigator of one National Cancer Institute (NCI) study, "The risk of breast cancer is not uniformly high for all women who carry a BRCA1 or BRCA2 mutation." [12] Findings suggest that carriers of one or more of three alterations found in higher proportions within these genes average a 56 percent chance of developing breast cancer by age seventy as opposed to 13 percent for the general population. What remains unknown is whether these alterations alone, or in combination with unknown genes or environmental factors, are the final determinants for the growth of cancer cells. Genetic defects in general are accountable for only 5 to 10 percent of breast cancer cases, of which, the majority of inherited cases are attributable to the BRCA1 and BRCA2 genes.

The *HER2/neu gene* is present in greater than normal quantities for between 25 to 30 percent of breast cancers. Over expression of this gene stimulates cell growth, and is associated with a more aggressive form of breast cancer. The latest line of attack is herceptin, a genetically engineered monoclonal antibody that locks onto the gene's protein receptor and slows the growth-promoting action within the cells. This magic bullet is approved for women with metastatic disease alone or in conjunction with chemotherapy. The next step involves clinical trials to test the drug's effectiveness in women with early-stage cancer. While herceptin has few of the common side effects of chemotherapy, it does have a downside—cardiac toxicity. A small percentage of patients, taking herceptin along with adriamycin and cytoxan (chemotherapy drugs commonly used to treat breast cancer), have developed heart problems. In a majority of these instances the situation is managed with medication.

These breakthrough discoveries are considered to be just the tip of the genetic iceberg, with major implications for future prevention and treatment of the disease via gene manipulation. It's important to keep in mind that unknown factors may increase or modify each woman's risk. Consequently, being a carrier of a genetic mutation in no way guarantees that a woman will develop breast cancer.

Lifestyle Risks

When it comes to reducing the likelihood for developing breast cancer we have no control over our genetic make-up or family history. But we do have control over our lifestyle habits, and this may mean the difference between getting, or not getting, breast cancer.

Tobacco Smoke: Smoking is considered a significant factor in the development of a number of diseases, including breast cancer. The carcinogens in cigarette smoke have been judged to have an antagonistic effect, especially in women who are genetically predisposed to react negatively to the chemicals formed when tobacco is burned.[13] If you presently smoke, there's no time like the present to stop. Begin on the road to improving your own health, and the health of your family since second-hand smoke also increases their risk for developing lung cancer and other medical conditions.[14]

Alcohol: Alcohol consumption has a deleterious affect on breast health. While suggested consumption levels vary from study to study all the evidence points towards minimal use of alcohol. One study found the risk increased almost 50 percent when two or more drinks were consumed on a daily basis (one drink is 12 ounces of regular beer, 5 ounces of wine, or 1-1/2 ounces of liquor).[15] Another study concluded that regular consumption of less than half of one alcoholic drink a day increased the overall risk by 50 percent.[16] For women taking ERT it's recommended that alcohol consumption be limited to one drink a day since even small amounts may prove detrimental. But for women who have had breast cancer, or have a family history of the disease, abstention is the way to go.[17]

Obesity: Obesity plays a significant role in the development of breast cancer. Researchers performing animal studies found that a lower incidence of cancer correlates with lean body mass.[18] While excess weight is detrimental at any age, it plays a particularly important role in the bodies of postmenopausal women most notably when excess weight is centered in the belly area. [19]

A 13-year landmark study, took place between 1959 and 1972, evaluating the relationship between obesity and cancer. Body weight, smoking habits, and the cancer deaths of over 750,000 men and women from 26 states were analyzed. Researchers concluded that, "after accounting for the effects of age and cigarette smoking, people whose body weight was 40 percent higher than average had an overall increased risk of cancer death" (33 percent increase in men, and a 55 percent increase in women). Overweight females had especially higher rates of breast, cervix, endometrium, uterus and ovarian cancers.[20] Along those same lines, an ongoing study of 95,000 nurses in the United States found that a woman's greatest chance of developing breast cancer comes after menopause particularly if she is between 5 to 44 pounds heavier than she was at age 18.[21]

In 1985, the National Institutes of Health (NIH) suggested obesity was a serious threat to the health of the nation, and the evidence continues to accumulate linking obesity with increased risk for breast cancer and a number of other diseases.

Nutrition

Living in one of the world's wealthiest countries, it's disturbing to discover that poor nutrition is so commonplace. Poor dietary habits have been implicated as a contributing factor for a number of ailments—heart disease, high blood pressure, adult-onset diabetes, and various forms of cancer including breast cancer. A number of years ago the phrase, "you are what you eat", became the mantra of a group of people who were given the appellation, "health nuts", for suggesting that certain foods and specific nutrients were needed to maintain a healthy body. Today the former phrase is even more compelling since a large segment of the population subsists on diets loaded with fats and sugars, and sorely lacking in nutritional value, all of which contribute to poor health and disease.

Environmental Risks

Early exposure to radiation, electromagnetic fields and contaminants in our food, water, and air were less likely to be recognized as contributing factors in the past, but recent evidence indicates that they may actually be contributory in various forms of cancer. A number of ongoing studies will hopefully provide a clearer picture of how these factors affect our body's genes and chemical properties.

Radiation: The significance of limiting both the intensity and exposed area during treatment with high-dose ionizing radiation was not always known. Over fifty years ago women subjected to fluoroscopy for the treatment of a collapsed lung, or radiotherapy in which the breast area was also treated, were subsequently found to have a substantially increased rate of breast cancer. [22] [23] In time, the medical establishment recognized this radiation risk, and began taking it into account when treating patients. Then, there are those women who as children, adolescents, or young adults were treated with radiation for Hodgkin's disease or non-Hodgkin's lymphoma. This treatment also increases the risk for breast cancer as the women age. As far as mammography is concerned, the significantly lower x-ray dose delivered by the modern dedicated screening unit is considered safe for its recommended use in detecting breast cancer.

Electromagnetic Fields: On-going studies of non-ionizing electromagnetic fields (EMF) continue to examine occupational and environmental exposure to electrical and magnetic fields around us. One component of the *Long Island Breast Cancer Study Project* (LIBCSP), a project of the NCI, seeks to determine whether a variety of environmental contaminants increased the breast cancer risk of women on Long Island in New York. As part of the LIBCSP, researchers are examining exposure to EMFs found inside and from power lines surrounding the homes of women diagnosed with breast cancer to determine whether the EMFs were a factor in their diagnosis. Many concerned women and their families await the outcome of this study, since this area of the country has a high rate of breast cancer.

Environmental contaminants: A number of chemicals have been studied to learn their effect on endogenous estrogen levels (this is especially relevant for women with estrogen dependent breast cancer). The list includes: pesticides used in food production; the end products found in car exhaust and cigarette smoke; chemicals used to grow and maintain golf courses and the lawns of homeowners; and industrial contaminants like electrical insulators.

Many studies have examined and found an association between higher levels of organochlorines and/or polychlorinated bi-phenyls (PCBs) in either the blood or breast fat of breast cancer patients.[24][25][26] Others have found no increased risk from exposure to organochlorines, like DDT, its metabolite DDE, and PCB's found in pesticides and industrial chemicals. [27][28] One study in particular demonstrated a synergistic effect that would result in breast cancer when certain organochlorines interacted in vivo experiments.[29] On-going studies will continue to investigate the effects of exposure to these contaminants and others.

The Environmental Protection Agency (EPA) recently issued a report on dioxin (a chemical derived from sources, such as medical and municipal waste incineration and paper-pulp production). The report labels the chemical a "human carcinogen." While stating dioxin emission levels have nose-dived since the 1970s it may still be a cancer threat to a segment of the population whose diets include large amounts of fatty foods, particularly animal products. The risk from dioxin varies within the population, but eating a low-fat diet that includes lots of fruits and vegetables would certainly be beneficial.

In addition, encourage your family members, friends, and neighbors to avoid the use of pesticides, and other items containing toxic chemicals, including wrapped food and microwave products covered in clingy plastics. Take the opportunity to contact your local and state representatives regarding your concern over suspected toxic materials.

PREVENTATIVE PROTOCOLS

World wide, researchers are working feverishly to find methods for preventing breast cancer, with limited success. For several decades women have been involved in a variety of studies seeking a prevention outcome. While there is no magic formula being advanced, a number of study results have demonstrated positive results.

Anti-estrogens: During the latter part of the 1990s Americans were hit by an avalanche of media reports concerning anti-estrogens—*selective estrogen receptor modulators* (SERMs)—and their effectiveness in preventing breast cancer in high-risk women. Tamoxifen, a drug given to women upon completion of treatment for breast cancer topped the list of newsworthy items. Initially, it was prescribed for a five-year period following adjuvant therapy to reduce estrogen levels in hopes of preventing a recurrence.

The Breast Cancer Prevention Trial (BCPT), launched in 1992, was undertaken to determine whether tamoxifen would also prevent breast cancer in women not yet diagnosed, but at high risk for the disease. In April 1998 banner headlines reported that clinical trials of the drug were being halted due to overwhelmingly positive results—approximately a 50 percent reduction of incidence for these women.[30] The medical community believed that such significantly positive results warranted stopping the study so that women in the control group could also reap the drug's beneficial effect.

But there is a downside to the tamoxifen success story—side effects. For women between 35 to 49 years of age the prevention benefits are great and the risk of serious side effects are minimal. Women 50 and older obtained similar benefits, but ran a greater risk of developing secondary medical conditions—endometrial cancer (cancer of the uterine lining), pulmonary embolism (blood clot in the lung), deep vein thrombosis (blood clots in major veins), and stroke. Therefore the appropriateness of tamoxifen in older women requires careful evaluation on an individual basis.[31]

The SERM, raloxifene, was originally administered to treat osteoporosis. In the Multiple Outcomes of Raloxifene Evaluation (MORE) trial the drug was administered to postmenopausal women diagnosed with osteoporosis but who had no prior history of breast cancer. After three years it was found to markedly decrease estrogen levels in breast tissue, and reduce the risk of invasive breast cancer by a whopping 76 percent. A side effect of raloxifene is deep vein thrombosis, but unlike tamoxifen it hasn't been found to have a stimulatory effect on the uterus.[32]

The STAR trial (Study of Tamoxifen and Raloxifene), begun in July, 1999 is continuing the process by randomly comparing the effectiveness of both drugs in 22,000 women. Eligibility requires women be age 35 and older, post menopausal, and at high risk for the disease. The recruitment goal for this study has yet not been met. For women interested in learning more about participation eligibility contact the National Cancer Institute listing in Appendix A.

Anti-angiogenesis: On Sunday, May 3, 1998 a front-page article in *The New York Times* generated great excitement by announcing the discovery of two anti-angiogenesis proteins that inhibit the formation of blood vessels, the means by which tumors continue to grow. Many cancer patients and their families frantically attempted to obtain these tumor inhibitors in hopes of finally securing a "cure" for their disease, only to learn that while *angiostatin* and *endostatin* have shown promising results in studies using mice, trials in humans for these two compounds had not begun. In 1999 the first phase of clinical trials for *endostatin* began with only small groups of patients. Phase I trials will determine the most effective dosage as well as discover any possible sides effects. As with other anti-angiogenesis compounds being studied in animals and then in humans, it will be several years before all three stages of the trials are completed, and only if proven successful will they gain Federal Drug Administration (FDA) approval, and subsequently be prescribed on a widespread basis.

Breast Cancer Myths

A great many women harbor erroneous beliefs concerning breast cancer risks, some of which have already been addressed. Yet, there remain a few commonly held beliefs that are largely false, and should be identified as such. By clarifying this data women will be less likely to blame themselves when diagnosed with breast cancer, and in other instances the truth will simply be ascertained.

Myth: Breast cancer is contagious, and is transmitted by air, touch, etc.
Fact: Cancer is not a communicable disease. Breast cancer is an abnormal growth of breast cells that result in a malignant (cancerous) tumor. Cellular changes in one woman will not cause similar changes in another woman.

Myth: The "one out of eight women will develop breast cancer" statistic means that out of eight randomly selected women one will develop breast cancer.
Fact: The one out of eight women statistic is based on a lifetime average for women living past age 85. Meaning, if a large number of women were followed over their lifetime to 85 and beyond, one out of eight of those women would be diagnosed with breast cancer sometime during that period of time.

Myth: Antiperspirants cause breast cancer.

Fact: Antiperspirants do not cause breast cancer. Rumors circulated claiming that antiperspirants and antiperspirant/deodorant combinations caused breast cancer by stopping the body from purging itself of toxins released through perspiration in the underarm area. It was suggested that use of these products caused the build-up of toxins, which when deposited in the lymph nodes in the underarm area, caused cell mutation and the development of breast cancer. The truth—perspiration is simply 99.9% water, sodium, potassium and magnesium, and non-toxic.

Myth: Underwire bras cause breast cancer.

Fact: The authors of one book stated that wearing an underwire bra was a major risk factor for breast cancer due to constriction of the lymphatic system in the breast area. The theory may sound plausible at first, but the authors didn't account for any of the other suggested or substantiated risks like age, obesity, environmental factors, family history, etc.

Myth: An injury to the breast causes breast cancer.

Fact: A blow or any other trauma to the breast does not cause breast cancer. As with other parts of the body, a benign lump (fatty necrosis) may result because the breast tissue consists partially of fatty tissue, which when injured may swell, become tender to the touch, and result in scar tissue when healed. Typically the symptoms disappear within a few weeks. This scar tissue can be mistaken for cancer on a mammogram.

Myth: Nipple discharge signifies breast cancer.

Fact: Many women experience nipple discharge, which has nothing to do with breast cancer. A discharge is not uncommon, and can be related to hormonal changes during puberty, pregnancy, or menopause. Nipple discharge is cause for concern when it's bloody, watery with a tinge of red or pink, spontaneous, and only in one breast. Even in these instances 99% of the time it's either a *ductal ecstasia* (benign duct damage) or *intraductal* *papilloma* (benign growth in the duct). Always check with your health care provider when any of these symptoms occur.

Myth: Painful breast lumps are not cancerous.
Fact: While the majority of painful breast lumps are benign, there are some instances where this is not the case. Check with your health care provider whenever a persistent breast pain or breast abnormality occurs.

Myth: Women with small breasts do not get breast cancer.
Fact: The size of the breast has no significant bearing on a woman's risk of developing breast cancer.

Myth: Breast-feeding causes breast cancer.
Fact: Breast-feeding does not cause breast cancer, in fact some studies have suggested just the opposite. While breast-feeding is not cancer causing, women who have in the past, or are presently breast-feeding can get breast cancer, but this is unrelated to the breast-feeding itself.

WHERE WE STAND NOW

We presently have no sure-fire solution for preventing breast cancer. Future chapters of the breast cancer story will undoubtedly provide the health care community with a greater understanding of all aspects of the disease, including new methods for prevention, better early detection methods, and improved and less toxic treatments.

In the meantime, we need to avail ourselves of the early detection techniques presently at hand—mammography, breast self-examination, and clinical breast examination—and take steps to reduce the controllable risks. Following chapters will show the way to accomplish this.

Chapter 2
A Complete Breast Health Program

Why is it that as women we are regularly called upon to minister to the needs of others? Take your pick—spouse, children, parents, siblings, grandparents or friends—any or all of them may at one time or another require our support. And, why is it we tend to assume responsibility for others even before considering our own needs? Are you one of those women whose long-range goal is martyrdom? If so, forget it, because taking care of others, especially family members, is usually expected, and in most instances likely to go unnoticed. Once you accept the fact that others have needs, and that when called upon you will more than likely minister to them, it would serve you well to add your own name to that list without admonishing yourself for being self-serving. And, what better way to initiate a plan for self-care than by utilizing the elements of a complete breast health program.

THE PROGRAM

A complete breast health program consists of three components: mammography; breast self-examination (BSE); and clinical breast examination (CBE), a physical examination of your breasts by a trained health professional.

Guidelines for the Early Detection of Breast Cancer

Ages 20-39 years • *Clinical breast exam every three years*
• *Breast self-exam every month*

Ages 40 & over • *Mammogram every year*
• *Clinical breast exam every year*
• *Breast self-exam every month*

American Cancer Society

Each segment of the early detection program should be undertaken at the ages indicated in the guidelines chart. Women with a family history of breast cancer, or other known high risk factors should discuss individual screening requirements with their health care provider.

DEVELOPING GOOD HABITS

While the suggested time for beginning breast self-examination is age 20, it's also appropriate for young girls in their teens to learn how to examine their breasts. Habits developed early in life are the ones most likely to be retained.

MAMMOGRAPHY: THE BREAST CANCER DETECTOR

Mammography screening is an essential part of a breast health program, and is presently the best means available for the early detection of breast cancer. Since the majority of breast cancer diagnoses are in women 50 and older, medical experts and the major scientific advisory boards agree that by age 50 all women should be going for annual screening mammograms.

However, some of those same experts express a different viewpoint when recommending screening for women between the ages 40 to 49. The American College of Obstetricians and Gynecologists (ACOG) and the National Cancer Institute (NCI) suggest women in their 40s, at average risk, get screened every 1 to 2 years with the proviso that they discuss individual risk factors with their health care provider prior to deciding whether to follow an annual or semi-annual screening schedule. The American Cancer Society (ACS) recommends women begin having yearly mammograms at age 40. Regardless of the screening schedule decided upon, the end result should be an initial mammogram by age 40 (African-American women and women at high risk should discuss with their physician whether to have a baseline mammogram at age 35 or earlier).

Reason for Mammography

The reasoning behind going for regular mammograms is based on two simple facts: 1) every woman is at increased risk for breast cancer as she ages, even without a family history of the disease; and the strongest argument for getting a regular mammogram is 2) its ability to detect breast cancer up to two years before it becomes palpable. With early diagnosis women have the advantages of both more conservative treatment and a better chance for survival. The illustration below compares the benefits of mammography to breast self-examination alone on both a regular and limited basis.

WHAT IS A MAMMOGRAM?

It's a low dose X-ray of breast tissue that screens for early stage breast cancers, and diagnoses suspicious lumps and nodules.

Size of Tumors Detected by Mammography and Breast Self-Exam (BSE)		
Average-size lump found by getting regular mammograms	1/8"	
Average-size lump found by first mammogram	¼"	
Average-size lump found by women practicing regular BSE	½"	
Average-size lump found by women practicing occasional BSE	1"	
Average-size lump found by women untrained in BSE*	1-1/2"	
Source: The Breast Health Program of New York		

Detecting a mass on a mammogram doesn't guarantee a cancer diagnosis. In fact, approximately 85 percent of all breast lumps are benign and are often the result of poor nutrition; smoking or inhaling second-hand smoke; alcohol consumption; excessive caffeine consumption; or hormones, with symptoms becoming more noticeable just prior to menstruation.

Cysts and *fibroadenomas* are the two most common benign breast masses. *Cysts* are moveable, fluid-filled lumps that may be tender to the touch or quite painful depending on their size and location. Women with cysts are often referred to as having fibrocystic breasts, "lumpy breasts", or the misnomer "fibrocystic disease"—it's a condition not a disease.

Fibroadenomas are smooth, marble-like breast tumors that show up clear on a mammogram. Most commonly found in women in their 20s and 30s, fibroadenomas range in size from microscopic to several inches, and should be monitored for change on a regular basis. Two instances where removal is advisable are when they grow large enough to distort the breast's shape, and when detected in middle-aged or older women to rule out breast cancer.

POSSIBLE PROCEDURES

One or more of the following procedures may be done to rule out a malignant mass.
- *Sonogram*
- *Fine needle aspiration biopsy*
- *Core biopsy*

In instances where the lump is not clearly definable a physician may schedule a *sonogram*, a non-invasive method of determining whether the lump is solid or fluid-filled. A technician performs this procedure using ultrasound equipment. If the lump turns out to be solid the doctor may want to aspirate it in the office, or send the woman to a surgeon more familiar with performing *fine needle aspiration*. During the procedure some cells and/or fluid are drawn from the lump into a thin needle syringe, and sent for analysis. Should both the sonogram and fine needle aspiration prove inconclusive then further scrutiny would necessitate either a *core needle biopsy*, where a piece of the lump or a portion of the breast tissue is removed with a larger needle, or a *surgical biopsy*,—almost always performed as a outpatient procedure—where either part of the lump or the entire lump is removed for analysis.

The breast tissue of menstruating women—whether young, middle age, or close to menopause—shows up denser on a mammogram than the tissue of postmenopausal women. This density is due to the abundance of milk glands, ducts, ligaments, and fatty tissue in the breasts and appears as cloudiness on the mammogram, making it more difficult for a radiologist to interpret. In certain instances a mass is seen on a mammogram, but cannot be clearly identified as benign or malignant. This opens up the possibility of either a false negative or false positive reading. Both situations arise more frequently in pre-menopausal women. A *false negative* reading occurs when it's decided that a breast lump located on a mammogram is benign and no further testing is done, leaving the cancer untreated. A *false positive* occurs when an area of the mammogram is read as abnormal although no breast cancer is present. As you might surmise, a false negative can result in inadequate treatment for a mass that calls for further medical attention. On the other hand, a false positive might necessitate a woman undergo one or more procedures in order to verify if a lump is cancerous when it's actually benign.

In spite of these failures, the NIH estimate mammography locates 75 percent of breast cancers in women in their 40s versus 90 percent in older women. Therefore, it's advisable to err on the side of caution. Have that mammogram!

Many women look forward to getting older and entering menopause, gladly relinquishing the burden of their monthly period. With the cessation of menstruation, women's bodies undergo a number of physiological changes. Some of these changes become evident in the breast tissue, including a decrease in density, and an increase in fatty tissue. The good news is these changes make it easier to differentiate between normal and abnormal tissue, and consequently increase the effectiveness of a yearly mammogram in diagnosing whether a breast tumor is present.

Unfortunately, a major problem exists—getting women to go for their mammogram, especially menopausal and postmenopausal women who are at greater risk. Women offer a variety of excuses to avoid going for a mammogram (you may even have voiced a few yourself).

WHY WOMEN AVOID MAMMOGRAMS

- *Health care provider didn't suggest it*
- *Fear it will be painful*
- *Fear of finding a lump*
- *Fear of radiation exposure*
- *Lack of health insurance*
- *Lack of time*
- *Lack of transportation*
- *Lack of childcare*
- *No perceived risk*
- *No family history*
- *Communication barriers*

Some of the obstacles listed are poor excuses for non-compliance. The remaining barriers can be overcome. Every state and county has clinics and women's health care centers (many affiliated with local hospitals) that will accommodate women dealing with a lack of health care coverage, transportation or childcare; limited financial resources; or communication barriers. While no one would like to hear those ominous sounding words, "you have breast cancer", the remaining reasons are simply invalid excuses for rejecting a protocol that offers the peace of mind women feel upon learning they don't have breast cancer. Alternative resources for information on free mammograms are county departments of health, state medical societies, local breast cancer coalitions, the American Cancer Society, the NCI's Cancer Information Service, or other health and cancer affiliated organizations.

Awareness of the age at which women are at greatest risk is not enough. The medical establishment cannot tell us who will get breast cancer—even women with known genetic abnormalities or first-degree relatives with the disease may never receive a diagnosis themselves. For that reason, we each need to do whatever we can to reduce our risk and increase our chances for early detection. Because going for a mammogram on a regular basis after the age of 40 is advantageous, it's clearly in the best interest of every woman to do so.

Going For A Mammogram

Now for a brief rundown on what to expect when you go for a mammogram. Though each facility varies the procedure slightly, they will usually begin by sending you to a dressing room to remove your blouse and bra and replace it with a cotton cover-up that opens in front. You will then be escorted into the room containing the mammography machine, and asked to remove one arm from the cover-up to facilitate the procedure. The radiologic technologist will then position your breast for the mammogram. The machine contains two parallel shelves, one stationary and the other moveable. The upper shelf is lowered to compress the breast tissue, and the breast is x-rayed. The same procedure is repeated for the other breast. Typically, two pictures are taken of each breast, one with the shelves in a horizontal position, and the other with the shelves oriented vertically. The entire procedure takes approximately 20 minutes.

MAMMOGRAPHY DAY

If you are uncomfortable with the idea of having to disrobe completely when going for a mammogram, wear a two-piece outfit.

The actual breast compression may cause discomfort, but fortunately the time elapsed for each picture is only a few seconds. Don't worry if you're told additional pictures are required. Occasionally, they are needed if the entire breast tissue was not visible on the x-ray, or if a particular area needs further scrutiny—*this doesn't automatically signal the presence of breast cancer.* Upon completion of the mammograms you may be asked to remain in the waiting room for a short time until the results are determined. Keep in mind, facility procedures and the services they provide vary. While some facilities provide the results immediately, others choose to notify patients by mail. A CBE may or may not be given. If you don't receive a CBE on the day of your mammography appointment, follow up and schedule one with your gynecologist or a trained health care provider shortly thereafter.

Mammography Checklist

Okay, now you're ready to schedule your mammogram. Before making the appointment be sure you're familiar with the following information.

1) The facility should have American College of Radiology (ACR) accreditation. All mammography facilities are required, through the Mammography Quality Standards Act (MQSA), to display certification from the FDA containing the facility name and the approval period of time. Certification means the facility has met the strict standards required for the equipment, record keeping, reporting, and the employees involved in the screening process. Prior to scheduling an appointment ask whether the facility is FDA certified, and look for the certification and the equipment expiration date on display.

2) The individual providing the mammogram should be a certified radiologic technologist, an individual who is properly trained to perform this task.

3) Many women—particularly those with cystic (lumpy) breasts—find their breasts are tender, swollen, and sensitive to the touch prior to menstruation. That's why it's advisable to schedule a mammogram 7 to 10 days after menstruation begins. Women on HRT should determine which days of the month are most appropriate, or ask their health care provider. While mammography may produce some discomfort, it shouldn't be painful. If the procedure causes sharp pain, don't hesitate to inform the technologist.

4) If you have breast implants it's important to advise the facility staff when scheduling your mammogram. If the facility won't accept patients with implants ask for the name of one that does. When arriving for your appointment, remind the staff that you require a technologist specially

trained to x-ray women with implants. The technologist will then be certain to x-ray as much of your breast tissue as possible.

5) A mammogram's clarity can be altered by any of the following—caffeine, powder, perfume, or deodorant. It's best to avoid caffeine for several days prior to your appointment, and not to use any powder, perfume, and deodorant on mammography day.

6) The physician reading the mammogram should be a certified radiologist accredited by the ACR. Your regular health care provider, or gatekeeper, is not necessarily the best person for the job. It requires someone with extensive training in this area with the ability to recognize critical changes. Having the mammography films read by someone with this expertise is especially important for women with dense breast tissue, where irregularities are more difficult to discern.

7) After receiving the results, if you have any doubt about what you have been told, don't hesitate to take your mammograms, along with a copy of the written report of the results, and go for a second opinion. Though facilities usually provide copies of mammography films, if requested, they're required to give you the originals. They may charge a fee for each film, which typically range from three dollars up to twenty dollars per film. (*Effective April, 1999 New York State legislation requires that all mammography facilities provide original films upon request. In addition, the facility cannot charge the patient for copies they make for their own files. Check your own state laws to see if there's similar legislation*). Keep in mind, if you're not given the results at the time of your visit, the 1999 reauthorization of the MQSA, requires that mammography facilities send women their screening results, written in layman's language, within 30 days or less. If an area requiring further scrutiny is identified you should be contacted by the facility within 5 working days or less.

> **REMINDER:** *It's best to take the originals when going for*
> *another opinion because the clarity of the films*
> *will be much better than copies.*

8) Once you begin having regular mammograms return to the same facility each year, unless you have a specific reason for not returning, like having moved since your last visit. When changing facilities, bring the originals of prior mammograms to the new location. These will be compared with the newest pictures, and serve to assist the physician in recognizing important changes in the breast tissue.

9) You can either schedule your next mammography appointment before you leave, or ask to be sent a reminder card. It's always a good idea to mark your calendar with a reminder when you get home.

Keep in mind that when circumstances demand it each of us must advocate for our own needs. If you are told your mammography results indicate no problem areas, but intuitively you feel something is wrong, take the films and go for a second opinion. If your health care provider doesn't cover costs for a second opinion (the majority of health insurance carriers do pay for a second opinion), check with your county Department of Health, and the other resources mentioned above for the names of facilities that provide either low or no-cost service. The bottom line is that you need to do whatever is necessary in order to receive the best health care possible.

BREAST SELF-EXAMINATION: PERSONAL CARE

Now we come to the second element of a breast health program, breast self-examination (BSE). Breast tissue is continually changing. These changes occur during the monthly cycle and pregnancy, while breast-feeding, when taking birth control pills and HRT, during menopause, and to some degree are due to the foods we eat and the medications we take. Any of these factors can cause fluctuations in the size, shape and texture of breast tissue. The most common changes occur in the middle of a woman's menstrual cycle when tenderness, fluid retention, and the appearance of lumps affect the breasts. It's not unusual for a woman to notice some variance during the month.

For that reason regular BSE, like mammography, should be done 7 to 10 days after menstruation begins to minimize the likelihood breasts will be tender or swollen. If no longer menstruating, choose a date and mark the calendar as a reminder (either the first day of each month or your birth date is a good choice).

> **REMINDER:** *Whenever you find a suspicious lump or notice a change in your breast, be sure to have it checked out by your health care provider.*

Try not to think of BSE as a search for that elusive lump. Each time you examine your breasts you'll become more familiar with how they look and feel, making changes more recognizable when they do occur. Initially, you might feel uncomfortable examining yourself, but remember it's *your* body, and the goal is to provide it with the best possible care.

> **REMINDER:** *There's no need to become obsessive about examining your breasts. When first learning to do BSE it helps to practice it more frequently, anywhere from once a day to once a week, just as a means of increasing familiarity with a part of your body that deserves special attention.*
>
> *When you feel comfortable with the process, once a month is all that is required, unless your physician suggests otherwise.*

Choose the pattern you're most comfortable with as long as you cover the entire breast area in your examination, *from the underarm across to the breastbone, and from the ridge below the breast up to the collarbone.*

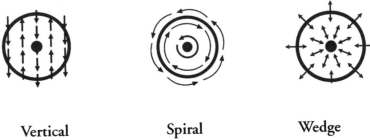

Vertical   **Spiral**   **Wedge**

VERTICAL ROW: Begin at the underarm area and work your way across to the breastbone in an up and down pattern.

SPIRAL (circular): Begin at the outer edge and move your fingers in a spiral toward the nipple covering the entire breast area.

WEDGE: Think of a clock. Move your fingers from the outer edge toward the nipple beginning at 12 o'clock, then reversing back toward the outer edge continue clockwise around the entire breast area.

How To Perform the Exam

In practice a good time to do BSE is just before bathing, or whenever you're able to find some private time for yourself. Let's go over the steps involved.

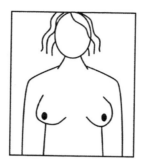

Step #1: Stand in front of a mirror with your arms at your sides. Look for anything that appears to be unusual for your breasts. Puckering or dimpling on the surface of the breast or nipple, scaling of the skin, any discoloration, or a discharge from the nipples are all signs that something is occurring within the breast tissue. Notice the shape of your breasts—you'll be looking for symmetry. Turn sideways towards the right and then the left to allow a side view of each breast.

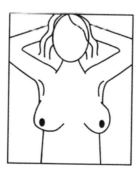

Step #2: Raise your arms and clasp your hands behind your head and press our elbows backward to expand the chest area. Look for any changes that alter the contour of your breast. Again, these would be swelling, dimpling, discoloration, and asymmetry.

REMINDER: *Each woman's breasts typically vary from slightly to greatly in size.*

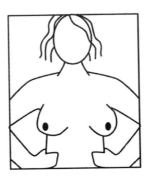

Step #3: Put your hands on your hips and bend slightly forward until your nipples point down. Check the front and side views for any change in the shape or contour of your breasts.

In Steps #4, and #5 you will be feeling for any unusual lump or mass under the skin. Breast tissue is composed of fatty tissue, glands, ligaments, and milk ducts so they won't feel absolutely smooth beneath the surface, but more like hills and valleys. A lump is unusual if you haven't felt it during earlier breast examinations—assuming this isn't the first time you're examining your breasts—and it now stands out against the texture of your breast. If something feels different to you, check the opposite breast for a similar ridge or bumpy area in the same location since it may just be part of your particular breast landscape. When there is a noticeable difference be sure to have it checked out by your health care provider.

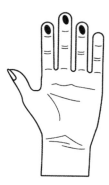

With the top joint of the middle three fingers (the padded portion not the tip) held in a relaxed position, follow the contour of your breast utilizing the pattern you've chosen. Holding the three fingers close together, move them in dime-size circles in an overlapping pattern of a finger's width.

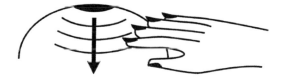

Use three levels of touch throughout each step of the examination: *light pressure* to feel just under the skin; *medium pressure* to feel the tissues of the breast; and *firm pressure* extending as far down toward the chest wall as you can without discomfort.

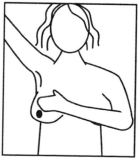

Step #4: Either sitting on a bed or standing raise your right arm. Using the pattern of choice thoroughly examine your right breast with your left hand. Change hands and examine your left breast. You may want to repeat Step #4 in the shower where your fingers will glide easily over your soapy skin, allowing you to concentrate on feeling for changes.

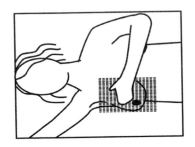

Step #5: Lie down and place a folded towel under your right shoulder. Raise your right arm above your head. Examine the right breast covering the area from the underarm across to the sternum (middle of your rib cage), up to the collarbone and down to the lower bra line (the bony ridge just below your breast). Repeat the process on your left breast.

For large breasted women: To achieve a better exam lie down, bend your knees, and roll toward the left so that your right nipple is pointing up. With right arm raised above your head and a towel beneath your shoulder, examine the outer portion of your right breast from the underarm area to the nipple between the area of the collarbone to the lower bra line. Without lifting your fingers, straighten your legs and roll onto your back and examine the inner half of the breast from the nipple to the breastbone. Reverse the process on your left breast.

For most women BSE takes about 15 minutes. If done on a regular basis, it becomes a habit—one that's certainly well worth developing.

CLINICAL BREAST EXAMINATION: THE YEAR-LY CHECK-UP

The third component of a good breast health program is a clinical breast examination (CBE) executed by a physician or other trained health care professional, typically the day your receive a mammogram, or every three years between the ages of 20 to 39. Since mammography misses approximately 15 percent of all cancer lumps, CBE plays an integral role in the program.

After taking a medical history, your health care professional should begin the examination by asking you to sit up on the examination table (the examination sequence that follows may vary slightly). Just as you did with BSE, she will be looking for evidence of puckering, dimpling, discoloration, nipple discharge or an inverted nipple (for a small percentage of women inverted nipples are the norm), or any other irregularities that suggest a possible problem. The areas above and below the collarbone and in the underarm areas are examined for lymph node enlargement, which can denote either an infection or a cancer that has traveled from the breast area. Palpation of each breast follows—this allows the health care provider to search for detectable masses. She should then ask you to raise your arms and press your palms together in front of your chest to contract the chest muscles allowing an abnormality to stand out. Finally, lying down with one arm raised overhead, your breast on the same side as the raised arm should be thoroughly examined with the procedure repeated on the other side.

If you feel your health care provider has given your breasts only a cursory exam, it's perfectly okay to let her know. For example, if your breasts and underarms were only examined while you were sitting up, you can suggest it be repeated while you're lying down on the exam table. It might even lead to inclusion of the reclining position into future CBE examinations of all patients.

When you participate in a complete breast health program rest assured that you are taking giant steps toward protecting your health.

ADDITIONAL SCREENING TECHNIQUES

Mammography is presently the best, and most widely available means we have for diagnosing breast cancer. But there are other screening methods that when used in conjunction with mammography can assist in instances where mammography alone is not sufficient. Combined use of mammography with these other diagnostic tools may aid in the early detection of breast cancer in women with lumpy or dense breast tissue due to a variety of reasons, i.e. prior biopsies or radiation treatment, and in other cases where further scrutiny is required.

Sonograms: Frequently used as a follow-up to a mammogram, a sonogram utilizes sound waves (in the same way as a ship radar searches the ocean bottom for objects) that bounce off a form and produce an image that can be read on a screen. Sonograms frequently pick up multiple masses (most often found to be benign lumps). When mammography detects a lump, sonography can determine whether it's a solid or fluid filled mass (cancerous or benign). Sonograms are most frequently used in cases of very dense breast tissue, extremely lumpy breasts, and for women with a family history of breast cancer.

PET Scan: The role of the positron emission tomography (PET) scan as an early detection tool is being examined in patients with dense breast tissue, fibrocystic breast condition, breast implants, or in other instances where mammography and physical examination are insufficient. The PET scan is also being evaluated in detecting the spread of cancer to regional lymph nodes and elsewhere in the body prior to treatment—offering women a non-invasive test that could allow many of them avoid additional surgery, including lymph node removal (a factor in the development of lymphedema, an accumulation of lymphatic fluid that can trigger numerous symptoms, including swelling, pain, etc. in an adjoining limb). Future uses of this test may also allow doctors to know early on whether treatment is working, or if it needs to be modified.

Magnetic Resonance Imaging (MRI): This test offers better contrast and image enhancement and is being studied for use as another means for diagnosing women for breast cancer. Researchers will assess the benefits of using MRI for patients with a genetic risk of the disease; for women with extremely dense breast tissue; as a follow up to regular mammograms when a suspicious area is located, and for examining the extent a cancer has spread within the breasts.

Miraluma (Sestamibi) Scan: This FDA approved imaging test provides doctors with another viable resource to use as a follow up to mammography when visible abnormalities or very dense breast tissue prevents an adequate viewing of the breast contours. It's a significantly improved imaging technique particularly for women under age 40, with extremely dense breast tissue. Performing the Miraluma test after an inconclusive mammogram may prove to be a valuable asset in securing an early diagnosis.

Quantum Well Infrared Photodetector (QWIP): This detection method recently received FDA approval. The QWIP, which also goes by the name Bio Scan System, is able to identify infrared energy (minute temperature changes) of blood flow in tissue. It works because cancer cells release nitric oxide that raises blood temperature as it flows around a cancerous tumor—similar to finding the hot spot in a fire. The measurement is then converted to a video signal that a physician can read on a monitor.

Devices like these and others that become available in the future, will only add to the early detection arsenal, and prove themselves capable aids in the battle against breast cancer.

Chapter 3
Good Nutrition Leads to Good Health

DIET OVERVIEW

Food is power. Food is capable of affecting how we feel, how we think, and how we act. At its best, food supplies us with nutrients that are capable of keeping our bodies running like well-tooled machines. At its worst, food deprives our bodies of the nutrients required to maintain good health, and in turn enables disease to run rampant.

A healthful diet is an essential component in the triad of diet, exercise and stress management. In the not so distant past the phrase, "you are what you eat", was echoed by individuals prominent in the then emerging self-health arena. Yet, for the most part their message was ignored. Throughout the 80s the number of people who heeded the importance of proper diet slowly increased, but poor eating habits tend to linger. During the 90s the public was on the receiving end of an incessant barrage of nutritional information through a variety of media sources, and on food packaging. Consequently, it is disappointing to learn that the general health of the nation has not shown more of an improvement. On a positive note, increasing numbers of women are exploring the available data to determine their nutritional requirements, and are seeking information related to disease prevention and lifestyle effecting changes like menopausal symptoms, suggesting that progress is being made.

What better way to begin the new millennium than with the affirmation, "I am what I eat." This statement is especially powerful when you consider that in addition to dietary and general health concerns, many women are also experiencing lack of control over other facets of their daily lives. By continuing to eat a nutritionally deficient diet they not only diminish their body's integrity, but also reduce their ability to deal with stress, a subject to be discussed in a following chapter.

So, what type of diet should be avoided? It's the diet the majority of Americans can't live without—loaded with fat, especially animal fat, high in cholesterol, caffeine and sugar, and low in fiber. Why do we love the foods found in this type of diet? *Because they taste so good!* Let's consider the typical fast-food meal consisting of a quarter pound burger with high-fat dressing, a large portion of french fries, a soda or coffee with milk and sugar, followed by a fruit pie or shake for dessert. Substitute a couple of slices of pizza or cheese tacos for the burger and fries, and the results are just as damaging. It's not unusual for a fast-food meal to contain all of the fat, most of the calories, and none, or few, of the nutrients our bodies require on a daily basis. Add this diet to a lifestyle that includes: tobacco smoking; a minimum of two to four alcoholic drinks per week; environmental factors, e.g. chemical carcinogens in the food, water and air; the use of hormones (ERT or birth control pills) and prescription or over-the-counter drugs, and we're setting ourselves up for dire health consequences.

Many of you might respond by saying, "well, people are living longer these days." But the truth is, a majority of the populace does so only because of medical support, at times an unreliable and lifestyle diminishing alliance. The goal then should not only be to live longer, but to do so as a healthy, fully functional individuals.

What Americans Are Eating

Societal changes have left their mark on how and what we eat. Many of these changes are in large part dictated by time restraints. As the number of female wage earners continues to rise, more women are racing the clock in the morning. Having to deal with time constraints most often results in an on-the-run breakfast for both the women and the remaining household members. Typically, a cup of coffee, and time permitting a roll or bagel are the easiest choices. In all probability lunch is eaten outside the home, except perhaps in cases where there's a stay-at-home mom. Junior high and high school age children, as well as adults, routinely make a beeline to the local fast-food restaurant on lunch break to indulge their taste buds. Many schools have cashed in on the trend and now serve fast food in the school cafeteria. In the past, dinnertime was the one meal of the day when the entire family was expected to sit down together. This custom is verging on extinction in most homes. As the kids get older and run off to other activities or to be with friends, and wage earners spend longer hours on the job, family meals inevitably go by the wayside.

Given the change in dining habits it's not surprising to see Americans making poor food choices. Statistics from the U.S. Department of Agriculture listed below tell just part of the sorry tale of the average American's yearly consumption priorities [33]:

53 gallons of soft drinks
23.5 gallons of coffee
24 gallons of milk

89 pounds of beef
47.8 pounds of pork
14.5 pounds of fish/other seafood

To start with, soft drinks and coffee (in most instances) are loaded with sugar, and both contain no nutritional value. The beef and pork, high in animal fat, are disproportionately consumed in relation to fish and other seafood, admittedly not everyone's favorite, unless fried, but certainly a food choice that should be eaten once or twice a week at the very minimum.

The NCI guidelines for a nutritionally sound diet, one that also helps reduce an individual's cancer risk, suggests cutting back on high fat foods, and increasing consumption of dietary fiber by choosing a greater portion of foods from plant sources like fruits and vegetables. Does this message sound familiar?

GUIDELINES FOR GOOD HEALTH

Fats

Fat intake is a hot topic these days. Most individuals concerned with losing weight are mindful of the fact that fat reduction is an effective way to achieve that loss. In addition, it had been proposed that consuming a low fat diet was beneficial in decreasing the incidence of breast cancer, giving women who chose this route a sense that their efforts were doubly justified. Recent findings from the Nurses Health Study suggest daily fat consumption of *less* than 20 percent fat is associated with *higher risk* of breast cancer! [34] Results from a study of this magnitude are difficult to ignore—information compiled on approximately 89,000 women over a 14-year period—but the bottom line hasn't been written. Another long-term study begun by the Women's Health Initiative in 1993 includes over 24,000 women eating diets containing 20 percent or less fat for up to 11 years. When this study is completed in 2007, researchers expect to have a clearer picture of the relationship between diet and breast cancer with additional factors, such as lifestyle and environmental contaminants likely to figure into the mix.

In spite of the recent study results there are still good reasons for reducing fat consumption to 20 to 25 percent of total daily calories. Young girls and adolescents who subsist on high fat diets tend to be overweight. Consequently, their bodies contain a surplus of fat cells—storehouses for estrogen. Since many breast cancers require estrogen to grow, girls who are overweight are encouraging the growth of cancer cells as they age. In addition, the greater the proportion of body fat, the sooner menstruation begins thereby increasing lifetime exposure to estrogen surges.

Breast cancer aside, prior to menopause circulating estrogen appears to have a protective effect in preventing heart disease in women. For postmenopausal women with greatly reduced levels of estrogen it's wise to consider the fact that consuming less dietary fat, especially animal fat, equates with a lower risk of heart disease, which for women in this age group is the disease with the highest mortality rates.

Getting to Know Your Fat Choices

Being aware of the type of fat you are eating can pay dividends since some fats actually convey nutritional benefits. The highly touted Mediterranean diet (rich in fruits, vegetables, and grains, but low in meat and saturated fats) includes the monounsaturated fats, olive and canola oils, rich in health promoting omega-3 fatty acids. These oils have an immune enhancing effect, and appear to produce a reduction in tumor growth. [35] Animal studies have found olive oil in particular is not the tumor promoter that corn and other polyunsaturated vegetable oils are. [36] Extra virgin olive oil should be your oil of choice since it represents the first pressing of the olives, and is subjected to less tampering than other varieties. The second runner up is canola. While canola oil has not been found to promote better health to the same degree as olive oil, it's still a good choice, especially if it's one of the organic expeller-pressed brands sold in health food stores. Whenever possible, supermarket brand oils should be avoided since they contain pesticides and other chemicals left over from the processing method.

Omega-3 fatty acid is found in a number of other foods. Multiple studies have confirmed the beneficial effects of adding fatty fish, rich in omega-3 oil, to the diet to prevent various cancers, including breast cancer. [37] [38] [39] Low breast cancer rates among the Japanese and Eskimos—consumers of diets low in saturated and polyunsaturated fats but high in the fish oil found in salmon, sardines, herring, mackerel and other cold water fish—attests to the likelihood that the fats in these fish act as breast cancer inhibitors. [40] Some additional sources of omega-3 fatty acids are flax seeds or flax oil, walnuts and wheat germ.

Polyunsaturated fats, such as safflower, sunflower, cottonseed or corn oils should be used in lesser quantities. These fats contain omega-6 fatty acids, which are unstable, can negatively affect the cardiovascular system, and produce oxidants and free radicals that damage cellular structure and promote cancer. While it's important to include some omega-6 fatty acids in the diet, if consumed in higher ratios than the omega-3's they can elicit a stimulatory effect on breast tissue, and over time may result in carcinogenic tumor growth and metastasis. [41]

Saturated fats like butter, cheese, and lard that are solid, or close to solid, at room temperature and the tropical oils (palm, coconut, and palm kernel) provide no health benefits, and if not avoided completely, should certainly be used in limited quantities. The same limitation applies to meat and meat products, which contain high amounts of animal fat.

Another class of fats, known as trans fatty acids, are found in small amounts in both animal fat and dairy products, but in most instance are obtained through a process called "hydrogenation", which transforms liquid vegetable oils into margarine and other solid fats used in cooking. These hydrogenated oils are found in many of the fast foods and processed foods Americans eat in large quantities, including most of the packaged bakery goods sold today.

Trans fatty acids to a greater degree than the other fats have been linked to a possible increased risk of breast cancer. One study of approximately 700 postmenopausal European women found that the women who consumed the most trans fatty acids were 40 percent more likely to develop breast cancer [42]. What makes these results even more disturbing is that, on average, the intake of these same fats by American women is *double* the consumption of their European counterparts, suggesting an even greater risk of developing breast cancer, along with the added possibility of elevated blood cholesterol levels. [43] The bottom line when considering any dietary fat, even the so-called "good" fats, is to limit daily usage since fat grams do add up.

Eating With Less Fat

Because fat imparts a distinctive flavor and texture, individuals may initially have difficulty modifying some recipes, eliminating others, and in general achieving the same sense of satisfaction when eating foods low in fat. In addition, they might be surprised to find themselves devouring large quantities of low fat foods in order to obtain the same sense of fullness once derived from their old eating habits. Of course then it becomes problematic to achieve any weight loss, or to maintain an appropriate body weight.

So what can you do? Begin re-training your taste buds by eating more health-promoting foods, such as beans, whole grain products, fruits, and vegetables that appease hunger and reduce cravings. *I can already picture the grimacing and moaning.* That doesn't mean you can never again eat a hamburger, a slice of chocolate cream pie, or any other food you crave. It does mean these foods should be eaten less frequently, and in smaller quantities.

The next step involves reducing animal foods to one serving a day or every other day, or better yet once or twice a week. Planning on eating a hamburger for lunch? Then consider a breakfast of hot or cold whole-grain cereal with fruit to start the day, and finish with a healthful portion of fish with steamed vegetables, a baked sweet potato and fruit for dinner.

Throw out the deep fat fryer. Fried foods may taste good and seem more flavorful, but should not be eaten on a regular basis. Use a non-stick pan and replace the usual oil, butter, or hydrogenated fat with a vegetable oil spray, or either chicken or vegetable broth. Broiling, steaming, and baking are preferred methods of food preparation (they may not initially be preferred by you, but give it time).

> **SYNTHETIC FAT SUBSTITUTES:** *Development of a man-made fat called Olestra has been hailed as the latest way for consumers to continue eating foods like potato chips while still limiting their fat consumption. The good news — this FDA approved fat is not absorbed by the body. The bad news — it reduces the absorption of fat-soluble vitamins, carotenes and phytochemicals found in fruits and vegetables — all vital in protecting the body against cancer (fat-soluble vitamins are added back, but not carotenes and phytochemicals).* [44]

One reason Japanese women have significantly lower breast cancer rates may be because they include less overall fat in their diet—they use animal fat sparingly in their recipes but consume generous amounts of soy protein, seafood, and vegetables. The fact is that when Japanese women adopt the American way of eating, which invariably includes more high fat foods, their breast cancer rates become comparable to the rest of the U.S. female population.

> **A SAD COMMENTARY ON OUR TIMES:**
> *Our Asian neighbors are strongly influenced by American dietary customs. With the proliferation of fast-food restaurants throughout Japan, China, and elsewhere in the Far East, we certainly deserve credit for ruining their centuries-long health-promoting dietary habits.*

So how about trying something new? Expand your culinary horizons. Dine out at a Japanese, Indian, Vietnamese or Thai restaurant as a way of acquainting your taste buds with a greater variety of food tastes and styles of cooking. All of these cultures employ a diverse selection of seasonings, grains and vegetables in their meals giving them a particular taste tradition without relying on excessive amounts of fat. Of course, it only works if you avoid menu items that have been altered from their original versions to accommodate American taste buds, or choices that are fried, or covered in heavy sauces—it's always best to inquire about the ingredients and the method of preparation prior to ordering. For individuals on a perpetual diet, an added benefit to reducing fat will be a greater weight loss and easier weight maintenance because fewer calories are being consumed.

> **THE CATCH TO EATING LOW FAT:** — *If you lower your fat intake, but replace the fat with too many goodies like no-fat desserts and soda, you will end up consuming an excessive amount of sugar and a large quantity of empty calories, and thwart any anticipated weight loss.*

Charting Fat Consumption

The procedure for determining the number of calories and the percentage of fat grams you want to consume to lose weight and improve your health is really very simple. Begin by tracking the present number of calories and fat grams consumed during a one-week period of time. Food and Drug Administration regulations require manufacturers to list the caloric content and grams of fat on food labels. If you have never examined a food label before, take this opportunity to learn more about what you're eating. For items without FDA labeling, e.g. fast foods, grains, multi-ingredient recipes, there are a number of inexpensive paperback books on the market that provide the count for individual foods by category.

Now you need to decide your weight goal, and the target percentage of fat grams you plan to consume—30 percent is the maximum advised. Begin your weight loss program by reducing your present calorie consumption by 20 percent. Drastic calorie reduction may seem the easiest route to achieving a quick weight loss—but it *never* works. This method only succeeds in increasing hunger, slowing your metabolism, and ultimately leads to failure. A gradual reduction in calories along with regular exercise, to pump up your metabolism, goes hand in hand (more on the exercise component in the following chapter). To ascertain the number of fat grams you want to aim for, multiply your decided upon daily caloric intake by the fat grams percentage decided upon, and divide the results by 9—each gram of fat equals 9 calories—e.g. 2000 calories X 0.25 (25%) / 9 = 55 fat grams.

Below are additional examples of typical daily caloric consumption, and the allowable fat grams, based on a diet containing 25 percent fat.

Average Daily Calories	25% Fat (grams)
1,200	33
1,400	39
1,600	44
1,800	50
2,000	55
2,200	61

With the multitude of choices available in the supermarkets and specialty stores, it's easy to achieve a reduction in fat by substituting the healthful, readily available low fat alternatives. Check out the examples listed below.

REPLACE	*SUBSTITUTE*
Butter/margarine	Olive or canola oil spray (for cooking) Low fat cream cheese, or fruit butter (as a spread)
1 Egg	¼ cup egg substitute or 2 egg whites,
Cream to thicken soup	Potato puree
Whole milk (2% or 1%)	Skim milk (for drinking) Low or fat-free evaporated milk(for cooking)
Oil for sauteing	Low sodium vegetable, chicken or beef broth Olive or canola oil spray
Mayonnaise	Low fat or fat-free mayonnaise Plain low fat or fat-free yogurt
Sour cream	Low fat or fat-free yogurt
Unsweetened chocolate	Unsweetened cocoa
Ground beef	Ground turkey
Creamed cottage cheese	1% fat, or fat free cottage cheese Low fat farmer cheese

Fruits and Vegetables: Powerful Allies

Consuming a wide variety of fruits and vegetables on a daily basis is essential for health maintenance. As an added bonus, they provide a potent source of antioxidants that protect cells from being damaged by cancer causing agents. And lucky for us most fruits and vegetables are practically fat free, rich in fiber, and chock full of nutrients like vitamin C, vitamin A, folate, calcium, iron, and potassium. Even calorie-dense fruits like avocado (yes, it's a fruit) that are high in plant-based fat can be eaten regularly, but in lesser amounts.

> **REMINDER:** *Eating different color vegetables every day ensures consumption of a good balance of vitamins, minerals, and phytochemicals.*

To the detriment of their overall health, most American's go year in and year out without consuming any, or only limited amounts, of these powerful disease fighters. [45] One survey from the NCI found that less than one-quarter of Americans eat the five daily servings of fruits and vegetables as recommended by federal health officials—consumption did increase from 19 percent to 22.7 percent from 1990 to 1996, not exactly what you would call noteworthy progress.

In most instances people rely on the same old vegetable standbys—carrots, potatoes, peas, and corn—or in the case of fruits—apples, bananas and oranges. While these choices are good food sources, broadening the selection makes menus more appealing to the palate, and increases the likelihood that your body will receive all the valuable nutrients required for optimum health. Fruits and vegetables have an additional benefit—they require little or no preparation.

Cruciferous vegetables like cabbage, broccoli, cauliflower, and brussels sprouts (assuredly not everyone's favorite, but certainly worth trying) are all members of the cabbage family and are potent cancer fighters. Phytochemicals found in these vegetables provide important antioxidant protection.

Nowadays an extensive variety of produce is available on a year-round basis. For increased anti-cancer protection choose organic foods whenever possible. Be adventuresome—try something different each time you shop, and before long you'll notice that your list of favorite fruits and vegetables has expanded considerably.

Fiber: The Great Protector

Dietary fiber serves several roles—1) it helps control an individual's food intake because the nature of fiber is to produce fullness, thereby regulating the amount eaten, and in doing so 2) reduces the risk for obesity [46]. The average American consumes only 10 grams of fiber each day, while the optimum goal to strive for is between 30 to 35 grams a day from varied sources. Even the typical American diet—high in fat, sugar, and protein—would be improved tremendously by an increase in fiber.

Good sources of fiber include fruits, vegetables, whole grains, nuts, seeds and legumes. The benefits derived from a high-fiber/complex carbohydrate diet include improved digestion, and reduced risk of adult on-set Type II diabetes (a disease with soaring rates among all age groups), varicose veins, arteriosclerosis and hemorrhoids. Insoluble fiber, such as wheat bran can be quite effective in lowering a woman's estrogen levels and effectively reducing her risk for breast cancer. [47] An added benefit of a high fiber diet is decreased transit time for stool to pass through the intestines, virtually eliminating constipation and the risk of diverticulitis.

ADDING FIBER

If your consumption of fiber has been minimal to date, it's best to:

1. Gradually increase the amount of fiber ingested in order to acclimate your body to the added roughage. Adding 5 grams a week until you reach 30 to 35 grams should do the trick.

2. Drink a minimum of 8 glasses of water a day.

3. Begin by eating small portions of potentially problematic foods, i.e. fruits, beans and whole grains.

4. If excessive gas is a problem, try one of the over-the-counter anti-gas remedies. Short-term usage is usually all that is required.

By simply beginning your day with a high fiber breakfast cereal you will be well on your way to meeting your daily fiber goal.

Three Important Choices

Two of the following choices have been stressed before, but bear repeating. First, with all this talk of diet changes avoiding obesity should be a primary goal. Postmenopausal women who gain a significant amount of weight increase their chances of getting breast cancer. Obesity is related to the number and size of the body's fat cells, which along with the ovaries and the adrenal glands produce estrogen. Under the right circumstances excessive amounts of estrogen promotes rampant cellular growth in the tissues of both the breasts and reproductive organs, resulting in cancer. So begin lowering your weight and your risk will decline too.

Second, alcohol consumption plays a significant role in increasing breast cancer risk. According to a recent study of more than 3,000 women ages 20 to 44 those women who drank a minimum of one alcoholic beverage a day, beginning in their teens and throughout their 30s, had an increased risk for breast cancer. By their 30s women who drank the most had the greatest risk—consuming 14 or more alcoholic drinks per week increased the risk by a whopping 80 percent. Logic would dictate that moderate alcohol consumption is the way to go. That means no more than two to four drinks a week. Some research indicates that even limited alcohol consumption increases breast cancer risk. Certainly, if you have already had breast cancer or are at high risk for the disease, abstaining from alcohol is the best choice.

> **REMINDER:** *Consumers are very accepting of foods with the "light" designation, believing that a "light" beer will not greatly increase their caloric and alcohol load. The fact is, not only might the alcohol in a beer increase a woman's risk for breast cancer, but it's probably being consumed in place of food that would be nutritionally beneficial to her body.*

Finally, minimize consumption of salt-cured, salt-pickled, smoked and barbecued foods, e.g. luncheon meats, hot dogs, and well-charred steaks and burgers prepared on the grill. Many of these items are high in fat, and contain chemicals like nitrosamine (a potent carcinogen), that trigger cellular changes, which can lead to various types of cancer.

Serving Sizes

Most people are confused about what constitutes a serving size. It doesn't help that they have become accustomed to today's typical portion sizes, which have grown by leaps and bounds. From 5-inch muffins and 6-inch cookies to 40-ounce soft drinks and double-decker cheeseburgers, our food intake has gotten out of hand. Is it any wonder obesity is on the rise?

Realistically, it's impossible for anyone to maintain a healthy body weight while consuming tremendous amounts of food. Learning the NCI suggested daily food guidelines becomes a reality check for most people because the majority of Americans have no idea how little food it actually takes to sustain a healthy body. The foods listed below add up to approximately 1,200 calories *(estimated caloric content of each item is in parenthesis)*. Adding servings in each category provides the appropriate number of calories to meet individual requirements.

Daily protein consumption might include:

1oz nonfat or low-fat cheese *(70 to 100)*
4oz broiled chicken *(140)*
8oz skimmed or 1% milk. *(80 to 100)*

One day's servings of fruits and vegetables should *minimally* equal 30 ounces or approximately 5 servings:

1 cup raw leafy vegetables *(25)*
1/2 cup cut-up fruit or 1 medium fruit *(50 to 80)*
1/2 cup cut-up raw or cooked non-leafy vegetables *(25)*
1/4 cup dried fruit *(100)*

> **Note**: *Only one-quarter cup of dried fruit is suggested. Foods with high caloric and/or high sugar content should be eaten in smaller quantities.*

Endeavor to eat seasonal and locally grown produce to increase the likelihood of getting the freshest products possible. When available, buy organic fruits and vegetables to reduce your intake of pesticides and other chemicals. Also, consider adding another four servings of fruit and vegetables, for a daily maximum of nine, to insure not missing out on any of the anti-cancer nutrients these foods deliver.

Whole grains, nuts, legumes, seeds and other fiber food selections on that same day might contain:

1 serving bran flake cereal *(70)*
2 slices whole grain bread *(140)*
1/2 cup cooked beans or peas (e.g. lentils, pinto beans, kidney beans) *(125)*
2 fig bars *(110)*

Keep in mind the calories can add up quickly. Eating foods from plant sources, unrefined and whole grain breads and pasta, brown rice, and beans several times a day is the best way to add healthful calories.

REASSESSING SHOPPING HABITS

Improving the quality of your diet by making certain it contains greater variety, and in particular more fresh foods, will probably necessitate revising your present shopping habits. But there is good news! For starters many high-fiber, non-perishable staples are available. Dried or canned beans, and grains—brown rice, oats, bulgur, barley and quinoa (keen-wa)—are just some palate-pleasing choices that warrant purchasing every few weeks. As an added bonus, leftovers from these foods are readily incorporated into meals on another day. For example, brown rice served as a side dish one night, becomes a low fat "fried rice" main dish another day with the addition of a diced, stir-fried assortment of vegetables, bits of meat, chicken, or crumbled tofu, and seasonings.

REMINDER: *When using a pre-packaged food or sauce, check the label for added fat, and salt, especially if you're on a salt-restricted diet.*

If you plan on eating five or more servings of fresh fruits and vegetables every day, it's wiser to buy them at least twice a week. When really short on time, purchase cut-up fruits and vegetables, but make certain they're fresh. Don't buy items with dried edges, or products that look like they've been exposed to the air for too long. It's always a good idea to have a package or two of frozen mixed vegetables on hand. Some brands of frozen vegetables include a packet of prepared sauce that serves to complete a stir-fried dish. Cut-up frozen fruits are readily available too, and can be eaten on their own or added to recipes to provide extra nutrition and flavor. Another simple short cut is accomplished when the most time consuming portions of a recipe are readied in advance (perhaps the night before), and then stored in the refrigerator until it's time to prepare the meal. Healthful eating may initially require spending more time making choices during visits to the supermarket and in meal preparation, but the end results will be worth the extra effort.

INITIATING DIETARY CHANGES

The idea is to make small changes in your diet over an extended period of time rather than radical changes overnight. Begin by examining your daily eating habits. Poor habits include frequently eating foods like bacon and fried eggs for breakfast, or a donut with a cup of coffee. Not eating any breakfast falls into that same category. Missing breakfast denies your body the fuel it needs to work at a high level of efficiency, and almost guarantees greater calorie consumption later in the day when you're less likely to burn them off. Frequently, women say "when I eat breakfast I'm even hungrier during the day than if I didn't eat anything at all." No doubt that's because breakfast consisted of food high in simple carbohydrates, e.g. muffins, bagels, or sugar-coated cereals that cause blood sugar levels to rise rapidly and fall just as fast leaving them hungry and tired.

Let's examine what might be a typical daily menu for the average American. The day begins with a cup of coffee for breakfast "to get going." Lunch consists of a sandwich (ham and cheese or mayonnaise-laden tuna are typical choices) accompanied by a soda (diet or regular). Dinner includes an iceberg lettuce and tomato salad soaked in Thousand Island dressing, a baked potato topped with two or three pats of butter, alongside a 8 to 10-oz steak and canned peas, followed by a dessert of cookies and ice cream or a slice of cake accompanied by coffee with milk and sugar. One day's meals like these supply too much fat, protein, and calories, too little fiber, and a limited amount of vitamins and minerals. Unfortunately, a dinner meal that size is usually eaten too late for complete digestion to take place, resulting in a bedtime accompanied by a full stomach. It's also likely that a variety of snacks are eaten between meals, and the proverbial "late night snacking" takes place in front of the TV.

After reading the contents of the typical day's worth of meals you should begin to have an idea of some of the changes needed—so let's explore how to go about it.

MAKING CHANGES

- *Identify daily eating habits*
- *Select unhealthy habits to be eliminated*
- *Seek out food alternatives*
- *Join forces with family and friends*

Begin by identifying your worst habits, and set about changing one or two at a time. It's a good idea to begin by keeping a diary of everything you have eaten (no cheating) for one week. Don't forget to include portion sizes. If you need help in measuring portions, purchase an inexpensive food scale. Most people are amazed to find out how much they are actually consuming. I know someone who eats a bowl of cereal in the morning, but uses the vegetable serving bowl that holds three or four times the contents of a regular size cereal bowl. A rapidly growing youngster might get away with this excess. But, if you think of it in terms of eating large portions of the wrong foods and multiply that by many times each day, the end result obviously will be weight problems and possibly dire health consequences.

> **PORTION SIZES**: *A common overindulgence is a simple bagel. The average bagel eaten today weighs in at 5 to 6 ounces, whereas a few years back the typical bagel was 2 to 3 ounces.*

Now you have to decide which foods can be eliminated completely, and those that can be replaced with low fat, fat-free and more nutritious versions. In the beginning you may find the process somewhat difficult, but once changes are initiated, and you stick to them, it will get easier—I promise. By taking small steps your taste buds will begin their "retraining" process. Foods you initially believed to be "yucky" or "weird tasting" may very well turn out to be favorites. Focus on replacing some of the high fat foods, especially animal products, with plant-based items, grains, and heart-healthy fish like salmon. An amazingly simple way to lose between 10 to 15 pounds over a year's time can be accomplished by eliminating calorie-dense, high fat between meal and late night snacks.

Begin keeping a "new food of the week" list. After sampling each new food, list the pros and cons. You may not like everything you try. Then again you may find lots of new and interesting items to include in your menus. In any event, it's always best to eat a wide variety of foods in order to receive all the essential vitamins and minerals to meet your body's needs and to avoid high concentrations of toxins found in certain foods. Enhance the flavor of food without increasing the fat, salt or sugar levels by incorporating herbs and spices into recipes. Don't be afraid to experiment. To expand your recipe repertoire check out a few of the excellent cookbooks available. Peruse some of the newer low fat cookbooks in your local library, and try a few of the recipes.

For individuals living with a spouse, children, other family members, or friends it's fun to divide up the planning and cooking chores. It's particularly important that children be allowed to participate in food preparation. Teaching children how to prepare nutritionally sound meals at a young age helps them to develop good eating habits for a lifetime. And by allowing them to prepare age-appropriate meals on their own you'll have less to do and more free time.

Are you among the approximately 80 percent of women who experience benign breast disease sometime during their lives? This is a situation, which in many instances can be controlled through diet changes—reduction or elimination of foods like coffee, tea (herb teas are okay), cola beverages and chocolate can help. A low fat, high-fiber diet that includes fruits, nuts, and seeds in limited amounts (excellent choices are walnuts, almonds, sunflower seeds, and ground flax seeds), fresh vegetables, and whole grains has been shown to eliminate or reduce this condition for many women.

THE SCOOP ON SOY

Soy products have risen from near obscurity to headline news, and for good reason. Whole grain, fiber, berries, most fruits and vegetables, flaxseed, and to a greater degree soybeans all contain plant-based chemicals called isoflavones. Sometimes referred to as "natural estrogen", isoflavones are much weaker than the estrogen produced by our bodies, and like the anti-estrogen tamoxifen they bind with the estrogen receptors in the breast and the uterus, effectively blocking absorption of the body's stronger version. Numerous studies link isoflavones to lower incidence of cancer in both the breasts and reproductive organs.

Additional benefits from soy in postmenopausal women may include a reduction of hot flashes, night sweats, and heart disease. Results of studies examining diet differences between Asian and American women suggest that, for the former, soy intake of between 30 to 50 milligrams of isoflavones a day, may be part of the reason why the incidence of breast cancer is significantly lower for Asian women.[49]

The health care community is divided on whether a woman previously diagnosed with breast cancer that involved estrogen positive tumor receptors, or a woman at high risk for the disease should be eating soy products. Some health care providers believe that because of soy's estrogen-like effect it should be avoided. If you are a breast cancer survivor, or are at high risk, talk with your physician about what would be best in your particular situation.

Since soy's boom in popularity, it's quite easy to find a complete selection of tasty products—soy milk, soy cheese, tofu, prepared main dishes, and even soy burgers and hotdogs are available in your local supermarket or health food store. These food items provide an effortless way to increase your intake of isoflavones (one-half cup of soy nuts, tempeh and tofu, or two cups of soy milk contain about 40 milligrams). Are you hesitant about eating soy or serving it to your family? Begin by incorporating one or two selections into the daily menu. Substitute soy for regular milk in pancakes or puddings, or enjoy a soy burger with onion, tomato, lettuce and other toppings of your choice on a sesame seed bun, but avoid the high fat dressings. How does a soy butter (this is a substitute for peanut butter not dairy butter) and jelly sandwich on whole grain bread, or silken tofu blended with a banana and strawberries into a fruit smoothie sound? Try some low fat grated soy "parmagiana" cheese in place of the genuine cheese—the taste similarity is astounding. As with any packaged food, be sure to read the label before purchasing a soy product since salt and fat contents vary. But most importantly, enjoy some soy.

DIETARY TIPS

With the emphasis on eating more healthfully, there are a variety of ways to boost the quantity and quality of the fruits, vegetables and grains in your diet:

- Snack on raw vegetables
- Serve soy meat-like substitutes, chicken, and fish several times a week
- Replace coffee, tea, soda or fruit punch with water, herb tea or real fruit juice
- Substitute the cream or half-and-half used in soups with potato puree
- Replace the oil in a cake recipe with pureed fruits or applesauce
- Store cut-up vegetables and fruits in the refrigerator for instant snacks
- Avoid menu choices containing fatty gravies, or cream sauces
- Enjoy whole grain breakfast cereals, breads, pastas, grains, and crackers
- Add fruits or vegetables to your favorite low fat cakes, breads and muffins
- Top your morning cereal with sliced fruit
- Flavor recipes with herbs, broth, or other natural seasonings
- Bring nutritious leftovers to work for lunch.

Use your imagination to create additional ways of giving your diet the nutritional boost and health-promoting essentials it needs.

Chapter 4
Exercising for Good Health

FACTS AND FIGURES

Exercise is a simple word that evokes complex feelings—from angst and anger, to confidence and contentment. Exercise can be a tonic for the body and the mind, yet for the majority of women it's just one more item jockeying for placement in an already crammed schedule. Historically, exercise is a natural phenomenon. Only in the past few decades has it become a separate entity and gone on to acquire a life all its own.

While participation in exercise programs has risen sharply, too many women still ignore their body's need for physical activity. For some women mention of the word "exercise" strikes fear in their hearts. The inclination is to picture someone like Jackie Joyner Kersey completing a heptathelon, or Debbie Austen teaching body shaping and toning—both women with bodies resembling fine-tuned machines. A very limited number of us are Olympians, star athletes, or built with nary a bulge in sight. Thankfully, few of us have the unrealistic expectation of reaching that level of perfection, and that's okay. So relax! There is much to be said for just getting up and moving your body. Walking, jogging, weight lifting, yoga, or any other form of exercise that increases your heart rate, tones your muscles, elevates your mood, and improves your general health is appropriate.

Numerous studies link regular physical activity to a lower risk of breast cancer. One study found that women who exercised an average of 4 hours a week since they began menstruating were 58 percent less likely to be diagnosed with breast cancer over the course of their childbearing years than women who did no exercise. [50] Results from a 14-year study of 25,000 pre-menopausal and postmenopausal women in Norway indicated that women who engaged in at least 4 hours of exercise a week lowered their overall risk of breast cancer by one-third. The added protection was "notable among lean women who were consistently active during their leisure time". [51] Even a woman's job can affect her risk. Findings from a study involving 5,000 women suggested employment involving moderate exercise lowered the risk, and that women in their 30s with jobs requiring moving around for the entire day reduced breast cancer risk by almost 50 percent. But, if you sit at a desk for most of the day, take heart. Thirty-something women who sat all day, but were physically active before or after work for seven hours or more a week reduced their breast cancer risk by 24 percent over women who were physically active less than two hours a week. [52] Results from these studies and others leave little doubt that regular participation in vigorous physical activity has a positive effect on risk. Two additional advantages derived from regular exercise are easier weight maintenance, and lengthened menstrual cycles that effectively reduce exposure to circulating estrogen—both benefits that increase in importance as a woman ages.

The fact is that for the majority of women weight gain is synonymous with aging. And the combination of turning 40 and gaining more than 10 pounds definitely increases their risk.[53] The effect of body size was evaluated in over 1,300 pre-and postmenopausal women. Regardless of their hip to waist ratio or body mass index (BMI) early in life, there was a subsequent increase in risk after natural menopause and/or after age 60 when they typically gained excess weight.[54] So initiating positive changes to shred those excess pounds sounds like to way to go.

For those of you who haven't developed the exercise habit take note, even unfit individuals who displayed only a moderate increase in fitness exhibited quite substantial health benefits. [55] It appears that exercise begun at any age has a beneficial effect. Consequently, there is no time like the present to begin your exercise program, and, if necessary, drop those extra pounds. As little as 20 minutes of exercise a day, a minimum of three times a week would be an excellent start.

> **REMINDER:** *If you are 40 years of age or older, overweight, have never exercised, or have a health problem consult with your health care provider before undertaking any new exercise program.*

THE AGE/WEIGHT RELATIONSHIP

It's a fact of nature that maintaining our figures becomes more difficult as we grow older. After reaching age 40 our bodies begin that inescapable transformation into what has in the past been referred to as the "matronly look". Just examine old family photographs. The majority of women—mothers, grandmothers and other female family members—years before the "youthful look" became de rigueur, were for the most part anywhere from slightly to greatly overweight, and in all likelihood didn't participate in any regularly scheduled physical exercise aside from their daily household chores.

Unfortunately, even today too many women are overweight, and avoid any form of exercise. The "fattening of America" is a phrase often heard. Lack of time, laziness, and the belief that it probably won't help are some of the reasons given for not exercising. For most women this downhill slide first becomes noticeable as they turn 40, or soon thereafter when they enter peri-menopause and begin traveling the somewhat slippery slope to menopause. Along the way they find that their weight and girth are climbing while their metabolism is taking the low road. As if an increase in body fat were not enough, there is accompanying muscle loss, due in large part to American's characteristic lifestyle—working at desk jobs, driving around in automobiles, and glued to chairs in front of computers and TVs. This muscle to flab exchange become evident during middle age but may actually begin taking place as early as our mid-20s—all the more reason to develop a taste for exercise early in life.

The question you should now be asking yourself is "am I presently getting enough exercise to maintain good health, and lower my risk of being diagnosed with breast cancer and other diseases?" Keeping in mind that exercise together with a nutritionally sound diet are essential for realizing optimal health. Once you have made the decision to initiate an exercise program, the goal of achieving an enhanced level of physical fitness will be accomplished by incorporating a variety of exercises into your weekly routine. As you will see shortly, this doesn't necessarily mean spending hours each day trying to squeeze a series of time-consuming exercises into your daily schedule. Truthfully, some of you may already be involved in physical activities that are deemed natural components of an exercise program.

BASIC COMPONENTS OF AN EXERCISE PROGRAM

A complete exercise program consists of three types of exercise—aerobic, range-of-motion, and strengthening, all necessary components for total body health.

Aerobic exercise, employs the large muscle groups on a rhythmic and continuous basis, and improves the capacity of the cardiovascular system by increasing the flow of blood and oxygen throughout the body. Activities like jogging, running, speed walking, bicycle riding, roller skating, and cross-country skiing are good examples.

Range-of-motion exercise, as the name implies, allows the joints to move within their full range of motion. This form of exercise goes hand in hand with stretching exercises. Joint mobility is essential, but is easily compromised without proper maintenance. Immobilization due to injury or pain reduces joint and muscle function. With range of motion exercises the elasticity and contractility of adjoining muscle groups is maintained. Stretching both arms out in front of your body, and slowly raising your hands overhead ending with thumbs touching is an example of a range-of-motion exercise.

Strengthening exercise increases the capacity of muscles to perform tasks, and while essential for women of all ages, becomes particularly important for women as they age. An excellent method for achieving your goal is strength training—beginning with 2 to 3 pounds weights and building up to 5 to 10 pounds or greater.

EXERCISE AND YOUR BODY

Regular physical activity has a lot to offer. Are you aware that in addition to reducing your risk for various forms of cancer, exercise lowers the risk for stroke, hypertension and osteoporosis, and assists in the management of diabetes and depression? Below are some additional ways exercise benefits both your physical and mental health. [56]

BENEFITS OF EXERCISE

- *Tones muscles*
- *Reduces fatigue*
- *Boosts energy level*
- *Improves self-image*
- *Controls appetite*
- *Bolsters immune system*
- *Reduces stress*
- *Lengthens time between periods*
- *Maintains cardiovascular health*
- *Decreases anxiety and depression*
- *Facilitates one's ability to fall asleep and sleep well*
- *Promotes weight loss and maintenance*
- *Offers an opportunity to share time with family and friends*

With all these possible benefits one has to wonder why more women aren't seeking the exercise fix. Are you still procrastinating? Then, to coin a phrase, it's time to take the ball and run with it. An excellent way to start your own program would be to undertake one or more of the exercises mentioned below.

> **REMINDER:** *The goal of exercise is better health, and that includes mental health. Pushing your body into an activity that stresses you either physically or mentally serves no good purpose.*

The exercises listed are only suggestions, there are many more to choose from, so let your imagination be your guide. Even activities like planting, weeding, or leaf raking in the garden provide excellent bending and stretching workouts. And let's face it, there are basic activities that as women we are most likely going to be doing—household chores. Yet even household chores can be considered a fun part of the exercise program—it's all in your attitude. Just keep telling yourself "I love vacuuming", "I adore cleaning the bathroom", "I feel so fulfilled doing the laundry". As you can see, a sense of humor is a real asset.

Sometimes the difficulty is in finding activities that best suit your needs and lifestyle. In part, choices will depend on how physically fit you are right now. Pushing your body into performing an exercise it's not yet equipped to handle won't be beneficial, and can in some instances be downright dangerous.

EXERCISE SUGGESTIONS

✱ *Running*	✱ *Cross-country skiing*	*Jogging*
✱ *Rowing*	*Stationary bike*	*Tennis*
Swimming	*Racquetball*	*Skating*
Weight lifting	*Low-impact aerobics*	*Walking*
✱ *Stairclimbing*	*Heavy housework*	*Hiking/Backpacking*
Leaf-raking	*Gardening*	*Dancing*
Bowling	✱ *In-line skating*	✱ *Power walking*
✱ *High intensity aerobics*	*Hatha Yoga*	✱ *Power yoga*

Now comes the hard part—selecting exercises that will work for you. If you think you will need moral support, choose activities that can be done with family members or friends. In addition, there are some general questions you should ask yourself when deciding whether or not to continue with an activity:

Sense of enjoyment:	Do I look forward to undertaking this exercise?
Immediate response:	Do I feel noticeably better after attempting this activity only once or twice?
Duration of the effect:	Does the improvement in how I feel last most of the day or longer?

The idea, of course, is to reap some benefits from the onset. In the beginning you may simply have a clearer head, and more energy during the day. As time passes, many of the benefits mentioned previously will begin to come into play.

If you're having difficulty reducing your caloric intake choose one or more of the activities (✳) that really bump up your metabolism—as long as your body is physically capable of handling the activity. These exercises elevate your heart rate, make you sweat, and boost your body's fat burning capability, especially when sustained for a minimum of 30 minutes. As an added bonus, your body continues to burn calories long after you've finished exercising.

One of your goals should be to intensify the pace to the point where your heart rate increases to a minimum of 60 percent and a maximum of 80 percent of its normal resting rate. To figure minimum and maximum target zones:

1. Subtract your age from 220
2. Multiply the result by 0.6 (minimum target zone)
3. Then by 0.8 (maximum rate for your age)

For example, a 40 year old would calculate target beats per minute (bpm) as follows:

220—40 = 180
180 X .60 = 108 bpm (minimum target rate)
180 X .80 = 144 bpm (maximum target rate)
Range = 108 to 144 bpm

Monitor your heart rate several times during the exercise period. Gently press your index and middle fingers against your inner wrist to check your pulse for 10 seconds, and multiply that number by six to get the bpm.

Are you working up a sweat just thinking about how much effort an exercise program is going to require? Well, stop thinking about it, take a deep breath, and let's get moving. I'll discuss three types of exercise that anyone can do. Each requires only minimum skill at the onset, but all three together will shape, tone, and strengthen your body. Discover what walking, weight lifting, and yoga can do for you.

WALKING FOR A HEALTHY BODY

Some people think that going anywhere on foot is a waste of time (sounds like they have scheduling problems), a silly idea, or simply an idea whose time hasn't arrived—for them. For others, walking is a gift that allows them to go someplace, or perhaps no place in particular because the simple act of walking is what they enjoy.

Walking is the greatest! Not only is it an effective tool for developing and maintaining good health, but if members of the health care community were asked to choose a single form of exercise that provides everything from a mental health tonic to an aerobic generator in an easy to access package, the answer would be walking.

BENEFITS OF WALKING

- *Needs no equipment, just a pair of comfortable walking shoes*
- *Requires only as much effort as you are willing and able to give it*
- *Fits into any schedule*
- *Appropriate for individuals of all ages, sizes, and shapes*
- *Brisk walking boosts the body's immune response*
- *Can be accomplished alone or with friends*
- *Reduces tension*
- *Race walking provides aerobic health benefits*

Getting Started

If all of those benefits are as good as they sound then there's no time like the present to begin your walking program. To start, you'll need to mark off a one to two-mile route. If there isn't a measured walking path in your neighborhood, use your car's odometer to determine a two-mile course, noting the one-mile point if you're only a beginner. If possible, measure out more than one route. This will allow you to vary the walk, and avoid the boredom of traveling the same course each time. If possible, refrain from walking on streets with heavy traffic to limit your contact with vehicles, and inhalation of exhaust fumes.

Begin by timing the one-mile walk at a comfortable pace. It might take anywhere from 20 to 30 minutes, but don't be discouraged if it takes longer or if you can't complete the mile. You're doing this for yourself, and it's only your starting point. In time, with repeated efforts your speed and the distance you are able to travel will increase.

As your body begins to feel more comfortable, gradually increase each session to 45 minutes or an hour. The method for making your body work even harder and increasing your heart rate, is to step up the pace. This is accomplished by taking faster steps rather than lengthening your stride—keep in mind that an train locomotive doesn't pick up speed by increasing the size of its wheel-base, but by increasing the speed that the wheels rotate. A reasonable goal is to walk a 14 to 15 minutes mile, three to five times a week.

> REMINDER: *Keep within your bpm range – don't push your body too far, too fast. If you're breathing heavily and perspiring but can still carry on a conversation you're within range.*

For another heart rate booster incorporate a hill or two into your walking routine. Walking uphill, to a greater degree than walking on level ground, involves the calf and the thigh muscles in the back of the leg, making stretching exercises particularly important (see exercises below). Be prepared, initially your muscles will feel a bit sore. Before long you should be as comfortable walking uphill as you are walking on level ground.

The Correct Technique

Make your walk a total body activity. Keep elbows bent at a 90-degree angle and swing them from the shoulder. Walk tall, with shoulders pulled back and relaxed, chest held high, head level, and chin held up in a natural position. Take long, smooth steps, without overextending the length of your stride. Keep the supporting leg (the one in back) straight as it carries your body forward, and allow your hip to rise and relax. As one leg moves to the rear, keep that foot on the ground for as long as possible before pushing off onto the other foot. After five or ten minutes of walking, your muscles should be warmed up.

Now would be a good time to stretch before continuing. While stretching won't build muscle or burn fat it's an essential part of an exercise program. By stretching you're preparing your body for peak performance, maximum flexibility, and a reduction in stiffness and soreness.

When your walking routine includes some hills, keep in mind that walking uphill requires leaning your torso slightly forward toward the incline, looking upward to see where you're going, and increasing the pace of your arm action.

Stretching Exercises

Achilles Tendon and Calf Muscles: Place both hands against a wall, or any flat surface, at chest height. Put one foot well behind you (about 26 to 30 inches). Keep the rear leg straight with its heel on the ground. Now, lean in toward the wall or surface, and feel the stretch along the back of your leg. Hold this position for 30 seconds. Repeat with the other leg.

Quadriceps*:* Place your left hand on a wall or other surface for balance. Reach back and grasp your right ankle with your right hand, and pull it gently toward your buttocks until you feel tension along the front of your right thigh. Hold this position for 30 seconds. Repeat on the left side.

Hamstrings: Stand on one leg and prop up your other leg parallel to the ground on a bench, or other surface that is lower than your hip. Slowly move both hands as far as possible toward the propped-up ankle. Hold this position for 30 seconds. Repeat on the other side.

Remember to begin walking slowly so your muscles can "warm up". End the session by moving at a slower pace again to "cool down". You may feel a bit stiff at first. If a joint feels sore, or if you think you've pulled a muscle, don't continue. Stop exercising for a few days until the injury is healed. If several days have past and the joint or muscle is still hurting, have it checked out by your health care provider.

Step By Step

How many ways can you think of to include walking into your lifestyle? I'll give you a few to start with, but you'll no doubt come up with some of your own.

There's a major benefit to living near an enclosed mall. Many malls sponsor walking clubs. They're especially conducive for exercising in hot, cold, or inclement weather when it's less desirable to walk outside. Some malls open for walkers as early as 6:30 a.m. permitting unimpeded exercising until the stores open for business. Of course, at any time of the day, particularly when it's not too crowded, you can walk to your heart's content and no one will stop you. A plus side to walking in the mall is all the money you will save by walking past the stores.

INCORPORATE WALKING INTO YOUR LIFESTYLE

- *Walk to the supermarket or other local stores*
- *Exit public transportation a stop or two before your destination*
- *Take the stairs instead of the elevator*
- *Walk with a friend*
- *Listen to your favorite music while walking* ✱ ✱
- *Explore local points of interest on foot*
- *Make walking a family activity*
- *Join a walking club*

Give It A Try

One of the phrases I hear most often is "I've got to start walking". But, if you follow the woman who said it to a shopping mall or supermarket, she can inevitably be seen riding her car around the parking lot in search of a spot close to the stores. Does that sound like something you might resort to? Then do yourself a favor—take a walk. If there is no precipitation, and you're not going to be carrying lots of packages, or will be pushing purchases in a cart, park at the other end of the parking field as far away from shopping as safety allows, and walk the rest of the way. It's amazing how habits develop after only a short time of consistent practice. Believe it or not, you may eventually feel cheated when you don't take the time to walk the extra distance. And remember, those short distances become miles over time. Just three 10-minute walks a day add up to 30 minutes of walking, which is just as beneficial as one 30-minute session.

> ✳✳ **REMINDER:** *Avoid wearing headphones in high traffic areas, like roadways. Or, lower the volume and move one earpiece behind that ear to enable you to hear the traffic around you.*

WEIGHTS AND YOU

In 1989 the U.S. Public Health Service Centers for Disease Control confirmed that less than 10 percent of all Americans undertake any form of physical activity that produces measurable physical fitness. This report notwithstanding, and discounting those individuals living under a rock since the news broke, most people are now aware that exercise is good for their health. Yet it appears that the majority of Americans don't believe it applies to them. Once upon a time women were expected to live with age-related body changes. The women may not have liked the idea, but they accepted it, and believed the gradual increase in weight, loss of height and strength, and the possibility of a potential broken bone or two was inevitable. For the past three decades there has been an ever-increasing emphasis on physical fitness. Beginning with the running revolution, followed by the aerobics mania, and for the past decade weight lifting, sometimes referred to as "strength training", has gradually increased its foothold, and might even be called by some aficionados the "exercise of the moment".

Many women begin experiencing health problems once they reach their 40s, 50s, and 60s—the most common one being muscle and bone loss. Yet it's possible to recoup a portion of those losses and slow or stop any additional damage. Once considered a male activity, few women elected to undertake weight training fearing they would end up looking like muscle-bound men. But over time and with encouragement from proponents in the sports, entertainment, and health care communities, weight training gradually gained acceptance. Growing evidence suggests that, regardless of age, women who undergo weight training increase both muscle and bone strength. For young women, indications are that if weight training is undertaken at an early age, expected bone loss will be minimal.[57]

During the past couple of decades the health and aesthetic benefits of weight training have drawn the attention of women from every walk of life and every age group. Encouraged by the possible rewards, women began to covet those much-touted benefits like improved overall body strength and appearance. Presently, weights are being lifted by young women searching for the perfect body; middle-aged women attempting to control the rapid "softening" of their muscles; and by older, post-menopausal women wishing to preserve or improve their bone strength to prevent osteoporosis, maintain their balance, or to simply manage their daily activities. Obviously, strength training's special benefits are important for women of all ages, regardless of their physical condition, and especially for women after the age of 50 when they enter menopause, and are more likely to be sedentary.

> ## BENEFITS FROM WEIGHT TRAINING
>
> - *Greater muscle mass*
> - *Increased muscle strength*
> - *Improved balance*
> - *Increased bone density*
> - *Greater endurance*
> - *Increased muscle to fat ratio*
> - *Improved mental function*

While aerobic exercise benefits cardiovascular fitness, weight training works its magic by increasing the body's muscle mass. An adult who doesn't strength train can anticipate losing between 5 to 7 pounds of muscle each decade.[58] That lost muscle inevitably turns to fat, resulting in a metabolic slow-down. But, replace the fat with muscle and you'll speed up your metabolism and burn more calories not only when working out, but all day long. Oh, what a lovely thought.

Finding A Trainer

While walking can be undertaken by most of us without utilizing the services of a trainer, beginning weight training under the auspices of a professional is advisable. Start by checking out reputable gyms and university or hospital affiliated exercise programs in your area where you can learn the basics. A good fitness trainer can be an asset in helping you to set personal goals, and in deciding which body areas need to be firmed up and redefined. Some individuals prefer using a trainer on a continuing basis while others will only require assistance in launching a program they can follow on their own. If cost is a problem, check with local gyms that offer limited-time specials and include the services of a trainer to get you started. Many town recreation centers, and local schools have facilities available where residents can work out for free, or a small fee. You might want to try the special membership at the gym and when it ends proceed to the community recreation center to continue your workouts.

By beginning a strength training program with the help of a professional, you'll learn the proper method for exercising each muscle group, and the correct lingo. Terms like lat pull down, leg press, bench press, arm curl, leg curl, military press, leg extension, upright rowing, calf raises, and sit-ups will all become as familiar to you as your own name.

Weight Training Suggestions

Whatever your age and physical condition it's important to begin slowly, and gradually increase the length of time and amount of weight used during each workout. Here are a few suggestions to follow when undertaking weight training:

1. Exercise a minimum of twice a week.

2. Choose a weight that allows you to do 8 to 12 repetitions of each exercise.

3. When performing an exercise avoid locking the joint, which can be weakened without proper support from the supporting muscle.

4. Begin with a weight that is 80% of the heaviest weight you can lift one time. For example, if you can lift 5 pounds one time, then 80% of that would be (5 x 0.80) = 4 pounds.

5. Move up by a pound or two when you can easily complete two sets of 12 repetitions.

6. Warm up with stretches for at least 10 minutes to prevent injury.

7. Exercise all the major muscle groups. Begin by concentrating on the large muscle groups in the shoulder, arms and thighs.

8. Alternate exercising each muscle group. Exercise the upper body one session and the lower body the next.

9. Perform each exercise slowly. Take 6 to 9 seconds for each repetition. Rest for a few seconds between each lift.

10. Inhale before lifting, exhale as you lift, inhale again as you lower the weight.

As far-fetched as it may seem at the moment, strength training can be a boon to your body. Whatever your age, imagine getting up each day with spring in your step, and the strength to perform the tasks you thought you couldn't possibly handle on your own. With an ever-growing selection of books, videos and local programs available for assistance, it's hard to find an excuse not to begin a weight-training program of your own.

YOGA: A LITTLE HISTORY

Webster's New World dictionary defines yoga as, "a discipline by which one seeks union with the universal soul through deep meditation, prescribed postures, controlled breathing, etc." For the majority of westerners seeking union with the universal soul is an alien thought, and the idea of turning to yoga as a means of staying healthy is as likely to happen as a tiger turning vegetarian. The remaining minority, who embrace yoga as a means of improving their bodies and minds, consider themselves lucky to have found a better way to take charge of their lives.

When yoga first came into vogue in the 60's most Americans looked upon it as a mystical and somewhat strange practice. Devotees emulated their favorite gurus by practicing the languid body poses (postures), sat crossed-legged while chanting "om", and burned incense—not exactly a sight most westerners could relate to. Western yoga practitioners were often hippies—thought by many to be "off the wall"—and other individuals who were not afraid to open their minds to a practice relatively new to the West. Like its multitude of followers over the millennium, they recognized the significance of the mind/body connection.

It now appears that after a long time in coming, yoga has arrived. Many Americans are hooked on yoga and have discovered for themselves its multi-faceted approach that leads to both physical and mental health. Yoga's components of meditation, breathing techniques and body poses have long been practiced in the East. Backed by evidence that yoga can provide aerobic benefits as well, it has now gained a niche in the U.S.[59]

Power Yoga: A Complete Body Workout

As Americans our hunger knows no bounds. When we're not hungry for food, we're consumed with finding new and better ways of depleting our bodies of its satiated fat cells, and firming our muscles, all hopefully accomplished in the shortest amount of time. To help achieve these goals Americans have finally not only recognized the value of yoga and made it a mainstream exercise, but have taken it to the next level.

The latest rage is yoga practiced as an aerobic activity, offering the same array of benefits as hatha yoga—improved stamina, balance, coordination, and mental focus. But, unlike hatha yoga, which emphasizes limberness and inner calmness at a pace more or less left up to the individual, astanga yoga, or "power yoga", is an intense activity incorporating yoga postures completed simultaneously with isometrics and meditative breathing. This is a demanding and challenging way to increase your heart rate, improve body strength and flexibility, and burn up to 300 calories a session. Power yoga is effective because it works several major muscles groups simultaneously. The program is not for individuals who hate to break a sweat. But, if you persevere, after as little as two months of twice-a-week intense workouts, you'll have achieved a new level of fitness. The focus is on performing conditioning exercises, while concentrating on breathing, understandably labeling power yoga "the complete body workout". The essential components of power yoga require a whole body commitment to the task at hand. An extra bonus is the development of mindfulness, the ability to focus with a single mindedness, which is beneficial in daily activities beyond the exercise room.

POWER YOGA'S EFFECT ON THE BODY
- *Toned muscles*
- *Accelerated metabolism*
- *Deepened breathing*
- *Improved flexibility*
- *Increased mental focus*

As with an aerobics class, power yoga is best accomplished with a teacher to help "keep the beat."

Hatha Yoga May Be the One For You

Some of us regularly participate in some form of aerobic exercise, and are seeking an exercise that is less body stressing. Others refuse to stand by the maxim "no pain, no gain" and simply want to pursue a less vigorous activity. Then there are those individuals who are physically unable to push their bodies as hard as power yoga requires. Yet they're all desirous of improved overall body conditioning. For these individuals hatha yoga is the way to go. Hatha yoga is the most popular form of yoga due to its litany of benefits, which are similar to those of power yoga—toned muscles, and increased flexibility, energy level, and mental focus, all possible from an exercise performed in a slow and gentle manner. For many individuals beyond middle age and well into their seventies, eighties and older hatha yoga remains a viable choice. Think of power yoga as the "hare" and hatha yoga as the "tortoise", and you know how that tale turns out.

A common mistake people make when beginning yoga is to allow themselves to be intimidated by postures that on first glance seem to require perfect balance, unlimited flexibility, and the body of a contortionist. Nothing could be further from the truth. When it comes to hatha yoga, it's possible to move slowly while concentrating on a movement, and still be rewarded with excellent results. Because it's an excellent way to wind down, for individuals on the fast track the benefits are even greater.

Hatha yoga can easily be done at home with the help of a video or one of the many books available, but you may want to get started by participating in a beginner's class. Communities everywhere offer yoga in their adult education programs. These classes are usually quite good, convenient, and inexpensive, with the added benefit of forcing you to set aside a specific day and time for participation. Many women find that while it's beneficial to practice yoga at home because of time restraints, it's more difficult to obtain the maximum results for the elements of deep relaxation and breath control. For those individuals classes are the answer.

> **REMINDER:** *Not all yoga teachers and classes are alike. Before signing a long- term contract, ask if you can join in for one or two classes to decide whether it's what you're looking for. Don't feel obligated to remain with a particular teacher if you aren't benefiting from the classes. After all, the goal is to reduce, not add to your stress load.*

Salutation to the Sun

Think of *Salutation to the Sun* as the yoga "sound bite". Did you say your body is feeling sluggish, and you want to get your engine going? Maybe you're feeling tense and worn out and require a brief respite—then *Salutation to the Sun* is the answer. To complete the prescribed series of postures a half a dozen times or less requires only a few minutes of your time, and a few feet of space. Perform the body postures slowly along with the correct breathing, and you'll calm both your mind and body. Completed at a rapid pace it will elevate your overall performance level, and get the juices flowing. An added bonus is improved flexibility regardless of the pace chosen. Traditionalists may practice the exercise early in the morning as a way to begin the new day, but it shouldn't be limited to only an a.m. tonic, it can be done whenever time and space allows.

Complete the twelve positions of *Salutation to the Sun* in order as given. Don't be intimidated by their description. Some of the positions will be easily accomplished—the remainder should be looked upon as goals to be reached over time. As a beginner, you may find it difficult to concentrate on both the movement and the correct breathing. Don't worry about it, first get the positions down pat, and the breathing technique will follow.

> **REMINDER:** *If any of the positions cause pain, or general discomfort, don't continue.*

FOOT AND HAND POSITIONS: Feet should be in the same position in numbers 1, 2, 3, 10, 11, and 12. Hands replace the feet in that same position in 4 through 9.

BREATHING: The correct breath for each position is indicated below.

Position 1: Stand straight with feet together. With palms touching one another, fingers pointed upward, and hands opposite the center of your chest. EXHALE

Position 2: Raise your arms above your head, locking the thumbs, with palms facing forward, and arms alongside your ears. Bend backward while looking up at your hands, with feet planted firmly on the ground. INHALE

Position 3: Bend forward, keeping your head between your arms, and place palms flat on the floor on either side of your feet. Keep your knees straight. Touch your face to your knees. EXHALE

Position 4: Keep your palms on the floor. Stretch your left leg out behind you, bringing the left knee to the floor. Keep your right foot between your hands, with the right knee touching your chest. Now, look up, tilting your head back slightly. INHALE

Position: 5: Without lifting your hands off the floor, bring the right leg back aligning the left foot with the right foot. Your body will now form an arch, with your head between the arms, and your heels stretching toward the floor. Now look at your feet. EXHALE

Position 6: In succession, bring your knees, chest, and chin to the floor. Keep your pelvis slightly raised off the floor. Palms should be flat on the floor beneath your shoulders, with your toes turned in toward your body. INHALE

Position 7: Lower your pelvis to the floor. Stretch your head, neck, and chest up, with head back looking at the ceiling. Keep your elbows alongside your body slightly bent so that the weight rests on your back. HOLD YOUR BREATH

Position 8: In one movement, tuck your head between your arms, and raise your body into an arch, as in Position 5, stretching the heels down toward the floor. EXHALE

Position 9: Swing your left leg forward between your hands, keeping the left knee touching your chest. The right leg is now extended back, with the right knee touching the floor. Tilt your head back and look up. This position is the reverse of Position 4. INHALE

Position 10: Bring your right leg forward, and straighten your knees, keeping your palms flat on the floor on either side of your feet (your arms will be alongside your ears). Bring your face to your knees, as in Position 3. EXHALE

Position 11: Keep your arms alongside your ears, lock your thumbs, and stretch your torso up and back, look at your hand, as in Position 2. INHALE

Position 12: Straighten your torso. Bring your arms down, and your palms together opposite the center of your chest, as in Position 1. EXHALE

THE "DROP IN, DROP OUT" SYNDROME

When it comes to exercise, the biggest problem we all face is the "drop in, drop out" syndrome. While many people are gung-ho about beginning an exercise program—drop in—they invariably find every reason in the book to stop exercising—drop out. It's amazing the number of replies non-compliance evokes. Some of the more common ones include: "I'm too busy", "I forgot", "I hate to sweat", "I'm too tired", "it's boring". Then there are those individuals who are truly creative, and come up with such memorable excuses as, "I couldn't get the knot out of my sneaker"; "the dog chewed up my socks"; and the one I found most bizarre, "my teenage son wanted me to hang out with him and his friends". My motto is "no excuses accepted", and I'm more than happy to share it with you.

Obviously, the idea is to begin an exercise program and give it a permanent role in your life. Most of us need a little (sometimes not so little) motivational push. Getting psyched to take time out of the day is not always an easy task. Below are a few suggestions to get you started and keep you motivated. The rest is up to you.

EXERCISE MOTIVATORS

- *Start off slowly*
- *Gradually increase the workout intensity and duration*
- *Keep a personal journal to chart your progress*
- *Set both short-term and long-term goals*
- *Reward yourself as you attain each goal*
- *Consider taking lessons*
- *Listen to your body*
- *Look for excuses to exercise more not less*
- *Choose activities you want to do*
- *Exercise with a friend of family member*
- *Vary the exercise to avoid boredom*
- *Make the activity fun not a chore*

Remember no matter what exercise you choose it shouldn't be something you constantly have to push yourself to do because we all know how that story ends. Think of your exercise program as a triad: 1) get started; 2) build up the momentum; and 3) stay motivated because the benefits are so great.

Chapter 5
Stress—The Good, The Bad and The Consequences

THEN AND NOW

When I find myself nostalgically recalling what it was like growing up two things stand out most in my mind—first, the less hurried pace of everyday life, and second, how well everyone managed without many of the "necessities" that presently clog our daily lives. The world has become more sophisticated in so many ways. Yet for all we've gained, so much more has been lost. As a result, far too many of us are strained by the conflict between "needs" and "wants".

Sophisticated communication toys and specialized gadgets clutter our homes and absorb most of our waking hours. More often than not these man-made products win out over the decision to put everything aside for even a short amount of time to enjoy, rather than seize the moment. Even our children spend far too many hours interfacing with invisible correspondents via computer. A large segment of the population live in single parent homes, where not only is a second parent missing, but once counted upon extended family members are only a memory. Is it any wonder that so many of us are unsuccessful in the search for that elusive element we believe will alleviate the stress filling our lives? We anxiously watch the news on TV, and read newspapers, books and magazines, anticipating discovery of that one special bit of information that will make us triumphant in our battle to cope, meanwhile being further stressed by much of what we see and hear.

STRESS EFFECTS US ALL

If it's any comfort, you can rest assured that stress is ubiquitous. But that does not in any way facilitate its control or preclude the fact that some individuals are more adept at coping with stress than others. Every day our bodies react emotionally and physically to both positive and negative changes in the status quo, which when not successfully dealt with allows stress to gain a foothold and remain a constant presence. The good news is that there are steps that can be taken to re-focus our energy toward management of those stress factors—the results being a sense of control, and a feeling of self-worth.

Stressful situations can be divided into two categories—"*major causes of stress*", which are life affecting changes often beyond our control; and "*complicating stress factors*" that tend to reinforce the former, and in many instances are controllable. Your particular situation may not be listed on the stress charts below, but that doesn't rule out its existence.

```
MAJOR CAUSES OF STRESS

• Death of spouse
• Change of residence
• Chronic personal or family health problems
• Loss of job
• Death of close family member or friend
• Divorce
• Marriage
• Pregnancy
• Caretaker of elderly parents
• Increased responsibility at work or home
• Mid-life changes
• Problems with loved ones
• Self imposed pressure to be perfect
```

```
COMPLICATING STRESS FACTORS

• Coordinating work and family schedules
• Dealing with traffic jams
• Lack of sleep
• Continuous interruptions
• Problems with a co-worker
• Deadlines, deadlines, deadline
• Fear of crime
• Bills to pay
• No time for own interests
```

For coping with major stress factors, or eradicating complicating stress factors determination alone often doesn't suffice. Many of us become overwhelmed when dealing with a particular situation, and have no idea how to begin to gain control. The first step in taking control necessitates recognition of which long-term and short-term events are having the most profound effect. That sounds easy enough. Unfortunately, being caught up in the moment, or weighed down by circumstances beyond our control can have a deleterious effect, and rather than allowing us to take charge of a situation, our emotions run rampant resulting in an accelerated heart rate, profuse sweating, and elevated blood pressure and blood sugar levels. Who hasn't at times felt like they were about to explode in anger or frustration, had a digestive tract irritated by rising stomach acid, or tightened muscles in their neck and back that caused severe pain? Unwittingly going through the day being bombarded by a multitude of stressful incidents ultimately wears down the body and allows subtle changes to take place.

Long term stress breaks down the body's immune system, and is linked to the variety of health problems experienced by many Americans today, including, heart disease, colitis, high blood pressure, migraine headaches, asthma, lowered resistance to colds and flu, and cancer.

A single significant life-affecting event, e.g. being postmenopausal, caring for aging parents, or the death of a spouse, within a five-year period prior to diagnosis, has been linked to an increased risk of breast cancer. [60] Focusing on adverse events without actively working out a plan of action or eliciting emotional support, can complicate a problem and lead to a reduced immune response and an increased risk of developing a disease like breast cancer.

DEALING WITH STRESS

We are complicated beings, each with our own way of responding to daily stress. Whether faced with a challenge, a repetitive daily scenario, or even a short-term change, while one person confronts it head on, another may feel overwhelmed and be devoid of an effective coping strategy. Here are three possible scenarios that might ring a bell.

1) Joan and Sally work for the same company, and are offered similar opportunities for advancement. Joan feeling confident that she can easily handle the job gladly accepts her offer and is looking forward to starting in the new position. Sally, fearing failure, turns down the job change, and is left to deal with frustration and stress-related headaches as constant reminders of her decision.

2) Lauren a young woman competing in a fast-paced, high-pressure job consumes a diet consisting mainly of snacks, junk food and meals snatched on the run. Lauren's stress from her job, combined with poor eating habits, leads to "burnout", evidenced by a long list of both physical and emotional manifestations.

3) Many of us look forward to going on vacation, and appreciate getting away from the daily grind. Others like Sheila, a high ranking business executive, thrive on being able to work long hours each day, and find sitting and reading a book, relaxing around the pool, or participating in recreational activities for long periods of time too stressful. Sheila finally decides to take some of the vacation time she has accrued, to unwind. After a couple of days of R & R, bored with the activities available to her, she has thoughts of an early return to work.

You may recognize and perhaps have even dealt with some of these issues in your own life. In that case, my question to you is—"how well did you manage the situation?" And if the answer is "not well", then your response should be, "where do I go from here?" Up ahead are some positive ways to defeat the *negative stress syndrome*.

Mid Life Consequences

The majority of women experience stress during mid life when a great number of changes are occurring, often at a rapid pace. Women in their late-40s and 50s are likely to experience high stress levels. This mid-life crisis occurs for various reasons—uncontrollable body changes, kids leaving or returning home, caring for aging and often ailing parents, jobs demanding too much time and offering too little satisfaction, and feeling they have not met their expected goals. These women, unlike their mothers before them, are often expected to be "superwomen". Add to this the prevalent attitude among the women themselves that they can, and will, handle all or most of what needs to be done, *and* do it well, leaves little room for failure. This need for perfection and the inevitable loss of control sets them up for stress that can, indeed, be devastating.

Symptoms To Watch Out For

It doesn't happen that one day we are stress free and the following day faced with some dreaded disease, with symptoms suggesting it's taking over our body. Both time and poor coping skills are powerful contributors to stress and its related disorders. Just how powerful a stimulus this combo is in undermining an individual's health depends on the present state of health, adaptability in day-to-day situations, interactions with individuals, and an individual's personality.

Two broadly defined personality types are dubbed "Type A" and "Type B". Type A's are described as ambitious, impatient, intense, competitive, hard working, and perfectionists. Type B's tend to be less ambitious, calm, fair, laid-back, and generally, at least appearance-wise, at peace with themselves and their world. The issue of control differs for the two types. True A's have the need to control situations and personal relationships, while B's have the tendency to "let the moment pass". As you might imagine, the former if unable to get a handle on their urge to control, are placing themselves at increased risk for developing stress related illnesses.

POSSIBLE SYMPTOMS OF STRESS

- *Chronic fatigue*
- *Weight gain or loss*
- *Change in appetite*
- *Shortness of breath*
- *Increased use of drugs/alcohol/cigarettes*
- *Back Pain*
- *Diarrhea*
- *Constipation*
- *Feelings of helplessness*
- *Change in sleeping or waking patterns*
- *Neck and shoulder pain*

- *Emotional outbursts*
- *Excessive spending*
- *Poor job performance*
- *Withdrawal or isolation*
- *Teeth grinding*
- *Heart attack*
- *Poor personal hygiene*
- *Headaches*
- *Indigestion*
- *Increased perspiration*
- *High blood pressure*

When under the strain of excessive and prolonged stress women may be left to deal with a long list of warning signs and symptoms that vary from person to person. Some of the symptoms listed are not typically thought of as stress related, but, clearly, stress is capable of manifesting itself in more ways than one can imagine.

Obviously, no one will be affected by all of the above stress signals and others not listed, but when symptoms develop, linger, and play havoc with day-to-day functioning dealing with them requires utilization of positive strategies to defeat stress's power hold.

REMINDER: *Some symptoms of stress can also signal the presence of other diseases or conditions. Anyone experiencing one or more symptoms, that linger, should be seen by their health care provider.*

HOW THE BODY REACTS

What happens to our bodies under stress? The body responds by triggering biological changes called the "stress response." [61] This stress response is part of what is termed the *General Adaptation Syndrome*, and consists of three stages.

STAGE ONE/ALARM: The body is jolted into reacting with an all-out push known as the "fight or flight" response. Either a single frightening event or long-term stress can promote similar body reactions. The adrenal glands are stimulated and send a surge of *adrenaline* and steroids throughout the body. This surge maximizes the body's ability to confront stress by redirecting oxygen and nutrients in the blood; increasing the heart rate, respiration rate, blood pressure, and muscle contractions; and decreasing gastric functioning, and abdominal and surface blood flow. Blood sugar (*glucose*) is diverted from the liver and released into the blood in preparation for increased alertness. Now the body is on full alert. In most instances this stage is short-lived, and the body returns to its normal state. When our ancestors were avoiding attack from charging animals the body's surging hormones played a vital role in their survival. Present day needs are not as great when we're facing a deadline or commuter traffic, but the rush is there just the same.

> **THE STRESS RESPONSE** *depletes the body of excessive amounts of protein, fats, and carbohydrates, plus vitamins and minerals whose stores cannot be built at an equally rapid pace.*

STAGE TWO/RESISTANCE: This marks the beginning of the long-term response to stress. Various corticosteroids, like *cortisol* continue to supply the body with energy to maintain a constant state of readiness.

Consequently, the heart works harder, the adrenal glands increase metabolism, blood pressure remains elevated, and muscle tension is unabated. During this period the damage is the greatest if the body is not allowed to return to homeostasis. While in this weakened state the body is less able to fight off disease. Cancer, heart disease and high blood pressure are diseases associated with long-term stress.

STAGE THREE/EXHAUSTION: Often referred to as the "burn out" stage. During this phase the body's ability to fight off infection and fatigue are greatly impaired. Energy levels are so low that even normal day-to-day functioning requires tremendous effort. This period heralds the take over of chronic illness.

The Breakdown

A typical example of a systemic breakdown occurs during commuter rush hour. Starting off late on a typical workday Mary focuses on arriving in a timely fashion when she's suddenly cut-off and forced to brake to avoid hitting an errant car. The alarm reaction takes hold, evoking anger toward the driver committing the action (this is a precursor to the infamous "road rage"), fear of having an accident, and general frustration. Hormones coursing through Mary's body trigger rapid heart rhythm, a sinking feeling in the pit of her stomach, contraction of arm and leg muscles, and formation of beads of sweat on her forehead.

In the resistance stage Mary's body attempts to repair the damage caused by the stress, until she's confronted by more close calls or traffic jams. In time she may become conditioned to expect problems on the road, causing her to automatically "tighten up" when beginning her daily commute. In all probability stress she deals with when off the road compounds the commuting tensions. Eventually, exhaustion takes hold and makes the development of a chronic condition a distinct possibility, which in and of itself further debilitates her body and immune system.

DAILY STRESS LEVELS

Identifying the causes and effects of stress in your life is the first step in a stress reduction program. Begin now by checking your responses to the following questions.

Read each item and check TRUE if it applies to you, or FALSE if it doesn't.

TRUE FALSE

1. I never have time for my own interests. _____ _____

2. I have no time for family and friends. _____ _____

3. I have no chance for advancement at my present job. _____ _____

4. I am not paid commensurately for the work I do. _____ _____

5. I am always rushing to stay on schedule. _____ _____

6. I am tired all the time. _____ _____

7. I am involved in a taxing personal relationship. _____ _____

8. I have difficulty delegating responsibilities. _____ _____

9. I can't say "no" to other people's requests. _____ _____

10. I am a procrastinator. _____ _____

11. I am unhappy with the direction my life is taking, _____ _____

12. I have trouble falling asleep at night.   _____ _____

13. I waken during the night and can't get back to sleep. _____ _____

14. I feel angry most of the time.   _____ _____

15. I eat when under pressure.   _____ _____

If you checked TRUE 2 times or less your stress level is low; 3 to 4 indicates moderate stress level, but action is needed to improve your quality of life; 5 and over denotes high stress levels that call for definite remedies.

COPING WITH STRESS

According to the American Heritage Dictionary "living is an active function", which is suggestive of a rhythmic forward movement. Let's, for a moment, call this forward movement "our path in life". The path you are on, like everyone else's path, has its twists, turns, and roadblocks that force you to stop and make choices. If a group of people who succeeded in getting past their own roadblocks were polled it's likely you would find they employed similar stress management techniques. Individuals who are the healthiest and in control of their lives, would be more likely to: 1) accept the fact they have a problem; 2) take the time to evaluate what should be done; 3) make the necessary changes; and 4) move with confidence past the obstacle impeding their journey.

Some women are simply undeterred by stress (we're not talking about the majority of women here). In spite of working, running a household, raising kids, and fitting in a daily exercise program that would humble the rest of us, they are enthusiastic, well-rested and full of energy, and when called upon can always find time for that one extra project. What's their secret for being able to do it all? In all probability these women are flexible, maintain a positive attitude, roll with the punches, set limits for themselves, know how to turn an unacceptable situation into an acceptable one, have found an outlet to relax and release stress, and refuse to deny their own needs. Well, if it works for them, it can work for you.

Every woman, no matter what her age, can benefit from knowing how to cope with stress. But where do you begin? First, by learning to recognize when stress is taking hold. If you're experiencing any of the early warning signs like tightness in the neck and shoulder area, back pain, nighttime teeth grinding, jaw clenching, and insomnia or erratic sleeping patterns you can rightly assume your stress level is elevated. Fortunately, in most instances these conditions are controllable. The second step requires uncovering the sources for these reactions. The best way to begin this process is to create a personalized *Stress Log* described in the four-step process below:

Step 1: For a period of one week to 10 days write down any situation that makes you angry, sad, frustrated, anxious, or in general causes a negative response to a stimulus.

Step 2: Record your response to each particular situation.

Step 3: Evaluate each item on a scale from 1 to 10 with 10 being the most stressful.

Step 4: Examine items rated 5 or above for a clearer picture of where changes will be needed.

The final step involves focusing on those issues that need addressing, and doing whatever is necessary to accommodate the changes. This is best accomplished by examining your Stress Log for recurring patterns. Did you have similar reactions during different situations? Are particular people or events repeatedly getting you down? What negative responses are you using? Are you avoiding certain situations or responses? Most of us give little thought to how we respond to daily situations, but seeing them in writing can be an eye-opening experience. Once you discover your stress patterns, and recognize your normal reaction during those times, you can begin a management plan. It won't happen overnight, but most women finally find the resolve to implement long-needed changes for the most damaging situations.

For some women it's not a simple matter, and assistance may be required. The truth is many of them have difficulty acknowledging a problem exists and asking for help. Without assistance they ultimately deny themselves the hoped for results. But it's unnecessary to do it alone. Seek out friends, family members, books on the subject, and local mental health providers—whatever it takes to make you whole again. After completing the restructuring of your life, and when you can finally meet the challenges of the day without feeling overburdened and unfulfilled, only then will you perhaps for the first time in years be able to derive pleasure and joy from each new day.

SAMPLE STRESS LOG

Negative Situation	My Response	Rating
• My boss often finds fault with my work	Angry that I'm unfairly reprimanded but rarely defend myself	10
• Carpooling often causes me to be late for work	Feel tremendous anxiety and guilt but aside from complaining to my car mates have not initiated any change	9
• I usually end up walking the dog	Resent having another chore	6
• Mary chose a restaurant I don't like for us to have dinner at on Thursday	Disappointed it wasn't my choice. I rationalized next time it would be "my pick"	3
• Tom and I frequently fight about the children	Furious that I'm continually being challenged, I usually end up with a headache or stomach ache	9
• Mom and Dad expect me to drop everything whenever they need something	I do what is expected of me, and end up with a tension headache and/or neck and back pain	10
• Accepted the PTA Presidency	Angry with myself for accepting the position, which will require too much of my time and energy	8

Meditative Relaxation

Let's for a moment assume you determined which stress-promoting incidents are causing the greatest damage, and have begun making changes to reduce or eliminate the most negative situations, but there are still occasions when stress gets you down and requires management—everyone has a hair pulling day now and then. Or perhaps even before you begin the stress reduction process you're willing to try a relaxation technique. Since it's going to be an ongoing and, in some ways, never-ending process, it's important to have access to various techniques for briefly escaping the tensions of the day. One of the most efficacious ways to get back on track is *meditative relaxation*. Interest in incorporating this tension reducer into overscheduled lives has spread, encouraged in large part by medical establishment "gurus" like doctors Dean Ornish and Andrew Weil, who tout the benefits of meditation, stress reduction, an enhanced immune system, and inner peace.

What makes meditation so special is its ability to minimize the drain on the body caused by the stress response. Anything that can effectively reduce the amount of circulating adrenaline and other stress-related hormones, lower blood pressure, release muscle tension, and decelerate your heart rate is certainly worth a try.

Meditation doesn't always mean sitting with a ramrod-straight back, crossed-legged in the lotus position, which for some people, including myself, is impossible. Many people prefer meditating while comfortably seated in a chair or reclining on a bed or floor. For others, a repetitive motion like walking or swimming, or simply taking a 20-minute soak in a hot bath can induce a meditative effect.

Two categories of meditation are *concentrative* and *mindfulness*. *Concentrative* meditation has an individual concentrate on a single word or sound (mantra), or focus on the inhalation and exhalation of the breath. Obtaining a personal mantra gained popularity in the 70s, with thousands of people often paying big bucks to some "smart cookie" for a few syllables they had to keep secret (I always imagined everyone was given the same mantra, but since revealing it was prohibited it was impossible to find out). Now we know choosing our own mantra or simply relying on the old standby "om" is perfectly okay

Mindfulness, or mindful meditation, as the name implies, allows the mind to relax and free itself from the thoughts and concerns of the day by permitting images to enter and pass through it without being contemplated. Its effect can transform how we respond to events, and even increase spirituality. [62] When practiced successfully, for as little as ten minutes a day, both types of meditation are capable of reducing the body's levels of anxiety and blood pressure, and enhancing immune function.

Systemic Relaxation

Systemic relaxation is another wonderful escape from daily activities. In as little as ten minutes it cleanses the body of all accumulated tension, and diverts the mind from the problems of the day. The key is to find a quiet place with no distractions. As a last resort some women have locked themselves in the bathroom and used the empty tub with a pillow for added comfort. Below is a body relaxation that can be read to you, or tape-recorded for playback whenever you feel the need to relax—preferably once a day. When having the relaxation read or taped, be sure the reader pauses several seconds between suggestions.......to allow time for implementation.

RELAXATION EXERCISE

All right, what I suggest you do now is to sit back in the chair, on the bed, or wherever you are...uncross your hands, and uncross your legs, close your eyes, and take a couple of very deep breaths. Take the breath into your stomach... make your stomach round and soft, and know that this is a time for complete conscious relaxation. This is a time only for you. This is not a time to think of the problems of the day. It is a time for you to relax as completely as possible. You will never be out of control. Everything that happens is well within your control. If my voice fades away, and you want to hear it, just slowly and gently bring your mind back to where you are. No matter whether you hear me or not on a conscious level, you will hear everything I say.

Now, you are going to travel in your mind down a flight of ten steps. As you approach the bottom of the staircase you will already begin to feel the tension

*leaving your body. Let's begin …1…… 2…… 3……4…… 5…… 6……
7…… 8……9…… 10.*

*Now, if it's comfortable for you…think of your left ankle, and your left foot,
and the toes of your left foot.….allow all the stress of the day to just drain out.*

*Now, think of your right ankle, and your right foot, and the toes of your
right foot, and let them relax. Just completely relax.…let all of the tension of
the day just drain out of your body.*

*Now, place your attention on your right shoulder. If there is any tension in
your right shoulder just relax it. Let all the tension and stress of the day just
run down your arm, and out of your body.*

*Now focus on your left shoulder. Allow any tension in your left shoulder just
pass down your arm and out of your body.*

*Continue to breathe normally and easily.….and picture your lungs as they
expand and contract. Feel your lungs as they expand and contract, and feel the
air going into your nostrils.…and coming out of your nostrils.*

*If you fall asleep that's okay. There is no way you can do anything wrong in
this situation…even if you fall asleep you benefit from what you are hearing.
You are in complete control…this is a time just for you.*

*Now, think of your right calf. Think of the long bone running from your
ankle to your knee. Think of how wonderful that long bone is, and picture it
in your mind's eye. Let all the tension and stress of the day run out of your right
calf.*

*Now, with your eyes closed, picture the word RELAX in large white letters
up in the sky. Now the word RELAX is just in front of your forehead.…. and
now inside your forehead. Concentrate for a moment on the word RELAX.*

*Now, picture your left calf…that wonderful long bone within your left calf.
Let all the tension and stress of the day drain out of your left calf.*

*Since the purpose of this exercise is to allow the tension and stress to just
drain out of your body.…if any part of your body does not feel comfortable…
just put your thought on that part of your body and allow it to relax.*

Now, picture your left thigh. Let all the stress of the day run out of your left thigh…and your right thigh. Think consciously of your right thigh…and allow the tension and stress of the day to run out.

Now, think of your whole pelvic area. Feel it relax. Feel the back part of your body against the chair, or the bed, or wherever you are. Be aware of the back part of your body…and feel how relaxed it already is.

Remember, everything you are doing is right…everything you are doing is perfect.

Now move on to the stomach area…let it all hang out. Allow yourself to feel at ease—completely relaxed. See the word RELAX just in front of your forehead…and, for a moment, allow the word RELAX to reside inside your head.

Now think about your chest and your lungs and feel them completely expanded… and feel how they feel when you have completely exhaled. Now feel your lungs as they expand and contract and feel relaxed.

Now think about the muscles of your face…all the muscles of your face…and your forehead. Let the muscles around your mouth completely relax. If your mouth falls open that's okay. If you feel yourself falling asleep that's okay. If you have lost the sound of my voice and want it to come back…then slowly bring it back.

Now behind your neck…and in back of your neck…just let it completely relax.

And now your left shoulder, and your left arm, and your left hand, and the fingers of your left hand…let them completely relax…allow them to be completely at ease. You can do nothing wrong…everything you are doing is just perfect.

And now your right arm, and your right hand, and the fingers of your right hand…let them all relax. All the tension and stress of the day is draining out of your body into the ground and into the chair, into the bed, or wherever you are.

Now relax the top of your head…and think about how relaxed you already are…and accept the fact that feeling relaxed is a wonderful way to be.

And now take a moment and continue to relax……feel the air entering your lungs……and feel them as you exhale………….

Now I am going to count from ten to one. When I reach one you will open your eyes, and you will feel at least as well as you did before we began.... and probably much better. Let's begin..... 10...... 9....... 8...... 7...... 6...... 5...... 4...... 3...... 2...... 1. You can open your eyes whenever you are ready.

Once the session is over, don't leap up into action. Give yourself a couple of minutes to savor the feeling.

Whatever meditation mode you finally choose keep in mind that while your attention is supposed to focus on a particular entity like your breath, a scene, or a sound it's bound to wander. Don't berate yourself just refocus on the meditation. Few people, especially beginners, are able to concentrate for long periods of time, and minutes can seems like hours when you're trying to clear your mind of all extraneous thoughts. Just allow yourself to enjoy the process, and the benefits will be even greater.

SELF-CARE TIPS THAT WORK

We all know what stress feels like. But each of us can also recall stress-free moments when nothing else mattered—lying back to watch the clouds float by, building a snowman with friends, running under the garden sprinkler or fire hydrant to cool off on a hot summer day. Can we really feel that way again? The answer is an emphatic yes. Here are a few self-care tips to help you focus on the goal of alleviating stress.

Exercise regularly. It can be any kind of physical activity—walking, hiking, bowling, tennis, bike riding—any leisure interest that effectively releases tension from your body, and burns off excess energy.

Eat Well. Make an effort to eat a well balanced and nutritionally sound diet. Reduce, or better yet eliminate caffeine, sugar and alcohol consumption.

Maintain friendships. Allocate time for friends. Share feelings with individuals you feel comfortable with and can trust.

Accept your feelings. Laughter has been called "the best medicine", but a good cry can be beneficial too. Both emotions release accumulated tension—don't deny yourself either one.

Learn relaxation techniques. Deep breathing, stretching, massage, and meditation are all wonderful ways to relieve stress.

Prepare for stressful events. Visualize yourself feeling relaxed and confident when anticipating stressful situations—and you will be.

Organize your day. Prioritize your daily goals and deadlines. Don't squeeze more activities into a day than you can comfortably manage.

Take 5-minute breaks. Every hour or so stop what you are doing and take a 5 minutes break to stretch, meditate, or do some deep breathing exercises.

Learn to say "no". Accept the fact that you have choices and use them wisely.

Get enough sleep. A well-rested body is better able to manage stressful situations.

Find a hobby. When immersed in an activity you enjoy the rest of the world just melts away.

Reward yourself. Anything that makes you feel good—a bubble bath, listening to music, reading a good book, going to the beach, gardening, visiting with friends, lunch at a favorite restaurant—reduces tension.

Whether you begin making changes to improve your health and lifestyle is ultimately up to you. But, remember there is no need for you to do it alone. Utilize the resources available to you, and meet the challenge. The end results will be well worth the effort.

Afterword

Okay, you done it, you've finished the book, and your head is filled with all those health-promoting ideas. Now don't let all that newly acquired information go to waste. Take the time to initiate whatever lifestyle modifications will benefit you the most to transport you on the road to optimal health, and reduce your risk for developing breast cancer. Some changes warrant minimal effort, like breast self-examination, getting a mammogram once a year, adding a few more vegetables and fruits to an already balanced diet, or taking a walk several times a week. Implementation of major changes like revamping your entire diet by reducing total fat consumption and introducing a variety of fruits and vegetables, giving up smoking, or allowing yourself the time for an exercise program—even if it's only twenty minutes a day to start—will require more time and greater effort on your part. Whether you succeed in achieving your goal depends on your willingness to participate in the process.

Take advantage of the resources found in the Appendix section. If you feel unable to do it alone, then don't. When necessary, seek help in getting started and continuing the process. Find a "buddy" among your friends and family who is willing to join you in following some of the suggestions in the book. Whatever you do, don't deny yourself all the rewards awaiting you when you finally achieve your goal.

About the Author

Joyce C. Smolkin, M.A., M.S. is Director of Breast Health with the American Cancer Society on Long Island working in the area of breast cancer prevention and early detection. She brings her experience as a breast cancer survivor to her job, her position of co-president of her local breast cancer coalition, and her involvement with various organizations that educate women and assist women diagnosed with breast cancer. She and her husband, Stanley, have two grown sons.

Appendix

The following resources are either ones I was familiar with, or simply felt would provide a broad base of information and support to inspire the readers to learn more about a specific topic of interest.

Many of the resources cover the same topics, but vary in their approach so choose those most likely to meet your needs.

The bottom line—use whatever resources will help you to reach the desired goal, and take whatever steps are necessary to maintain good health because it's your most valuable asset.

Appendix A

Breast Health Resources

American Cancer Society (ACS)
National Home Office:
1599 Clifton Road NE
Atlanta, GA 30329-4251
Toll Free Number: 1-800-ACS-2345
Web Site: *www.cancer.org*
Business Hours: 24 hours a day, 7 days a week
Services: Cancer information specialists provide information and publications, and connect callers with regional offices for information on community services and breast health programs presented by ACS trained volunteers. Information is also available on local American College of Radiology (ACR) accredited mammography-screening centers. Log onto ACS's website for the Cancer Resource Center and Cancer Survivors Network.

Susan G. Komen Breast Cancer Foundation
5005 LBJ Freeway—Suite 250
Dallas, TX 75244
Toll Free Hotline: 1-800-IM-AWARE (1-800-462-9273)
Website: *www.komen.org*
Services: Trained volunteers, many breast cancer survivors, offer information and support in English and Spanish. The foundation's focus is education, research, screening, and treatment.

National Alliance of Breast Cancer Organizations (NABCO)
9 East 37th Street, 10th floor
New York, NY 10016
Telephone: 1-888-80-NABCO (1-888-806-2226) or 1-212-719-0154
Website: *www.nabco.org*
Services: Answers questions regarding risk, detection and treatment of breast cancer. Provides resource information, and links to breast cancer and other health related web sites.

National Cancer Institute (NCI)
Cancer Information Center
31 Center Drive MSC 2580
Bethesda, MD 20892-2580
Toll Free Number: 1-800-4-CANCER—*Cancer Information Service*
Web Site: *www.nci.nih.gov*
Business Hours: 9:00 AM—4:30 PM, Monday—Friday
Services: Call center provides information and publications on cancer research including information on the STAR trial mentioned in Chapter 1, diagnosis and treatment. Callers can be connected to a regional office for information on community services. Here's an opportunity to speak directly with a cancer specialist capable of making appropriate referrals. Information is also provided on local American College of Radiology (ACR) accredited mammography-screening centers.

Book and Websites

The Boston Women's Health Book Collective, *Our Bodies, Ourselves for the New Century: A Book by and for Women* (New York: Touchtone Books, 1998). Every woman should read America's foremost resource and educational guide on women's health care and life issues—a direct result of the women's movement.

Karen J. Carlson, M.D., Stephanie A. Eisenstat, M.D. and Terra Ziporyn, Ph.D, *The Harvard Guide to Women's Health (Harvard University Press Reference Library)* (Boston, MA: Harvard University Press, 1997 paperback). A comprehensive resource for women and their families that covers an amalgam of health issues alphabetically arranged, cross-referenced and indexed.

Susan Love, M.D. with Karen Lindsey, *Dr. Susan Love's Breast Book* (New York: Perseus Books, 1999). Everything you ever wanted to know about breasts and their care. Includes pertinent information on breast cancer prevention, risks, conditions, diagnosis, treatment, and controversies.

Christiane Northrup, M.D., *Women's Bodies, Women's Wisdom: Creating Physical and Emotional Health and Healing* (New York: Bantam Books, 1998) A book that will enlighten and empower the reader with information on women's health issues utilizing both allopathic treatment and complementary therapies. A must read.

Anthony R. Scialli, M.D. Editor-in-Chief, *The National Women's Health Resource Center's Book of Women's Health: Your Comprehensive Guide to Health and Well-Being* (New York: William Morrow & Company, 1999) General guide for women's health maintenance, including special health concerns.

Nancy Snyderman, M.D. *Dr. Nancy Snyderman's Guide to Good Health: What Every Forty-Plus Woman Should Know About Her Changing Body* (New York: Harvest Books, 1996) Details issues relevant to women who have entered or are approaching the time in their lives when a multitude of changes occur. This is an excellent resource.

Lila A. Wallis M.D. with Marian Betancourt, *The Whole Woman: Take Charge of Your Health in Every Phase of Your Life* (New York: Avon Books, 1999) Details the four phases of a woman's life (adolescence, adulthood, perimenopause and postmenopause) and the inherent health risks and requirements during each phase.

www.womentowomen.com is a top-notch site for women ages 18 to 80 plus that provides access to information related to women's health brought to you by Dr. Christiane Northrup and her associates. Provides resources on both conventional medicine and alternative health care.

www.women.com/health/breastcancer is the equivalent of Breast Health 101. The site offers basic facts plus information on self-examination, steps to increase awareness and reduce risk, and answers to frequently asked questions.

www.allhealth.com/breastcancer provides women's health information similar to that found at www.womentowomen.com.

www.celebratinglife.org is the site for foundation of the same name that seeks to increase breast cancer awareness for African-American women and other women of color.

www.phenomenalwomen.com/breast-cancer is a site worth exploring. It contains a vast collection of information on prevention, organizations and institutions, awareness, treatment, resources and much more. You can send your friends a personalized breast cancer awareness postcard.

www.tricaresw.af.mil/breastcd/breast_cd_lg.htm is the Interactive Breast Cancer Web Site. Here's an opportunity to view three on-line videos on breast self-examination, clinical breast examination and mammography that explain what transpires during each procedure. There's also a personal breast cancer risk analysis you can complete. Check it out.

Appendix B

Nutrition Resources

National Center for Nutrition and Dietetics (NCND)
The hotline at 1-800-366-1655 will connect the caller to a registered dietitian who can answer nutrition and food questions. Monthly nutrition messages and fact sheets are available with practical and creative suggestions for healthful eating.

Books and Websites

Phyllis A. Balch and James F. Balch, M.D., *Prescription for Dietary Wellness: Using Foods to Heal* (Garden City, NY: Avery Publishing, 1992) This book is chock full of super tips for healthful eating along with health-promoting dietary guidelines.

Jean Carper, *Food: Your Miracle Medicine: How Food Can Prevent and Cure Over 100 Symptoms and Problems* (New York: Harper Paperbacks, 1998) Practical advice on how and which foods prevent and remedy common maladies.

Annemarie Colbin, *Food and Healing* (New York: Ballantine Books, 1996) Focuses on the role of diet and how it affects overall health.

Ann Louise Gittleman with J. Lynne Dodson, *Super Nutrition for Women: a Food-Wise Guide for Health, Beauty, Energy and Immunity* (New York: Bantam Books, 1991) A guide that assists women in improving their health, immunity and overall well being.

Nikki & David Goldbeck, *The Healthiest Diet In The World* (New York: Dutton, 1998) The authors offer a personalized diet for individuals based on information they gathered during their 25 years of work in the area of food and nutrition. This tome includes some great healthful recipes.

Sari Harrar, and Barbara Loecher, *Food & You: A Woman's Guide* (Emmanus, PA: Rodale Press, 1998) Information about foods we typically eat, foods we should be eating, and maladies that can affect us.

J. Robert Hatherill, *Eat to Beat Cancer* (Los Angeles, CA: Renaissance Books, 1998) Guide for utilizing foods in an easily adapted cancer risk-reducing regime.

Susan M. Kleiner, and Karen Friedman-Kester, *The Be Healthier Feel Stronger Vegetarian Cookbook* (Foster City, CA: IDG Books, 1997) Offers nutrient-packed recipes and dietary suggestions to support a physically active vegetarian lifestyle.

Carol Ann Rinzler, *Nutrition for Dummies* (Foster City, CA: IDG Books, 1999) A fact-filled tome on nutrition that includes information on foods that keep us healthy, natural vs. processed, food and medicine interactions and much more. This is an excellent resource.

Artemis P. Simopoulos, M.D. and Jo Robinson, *Omega Diet: The Lifesaving Nutritional Program Based on the Diet of the Island of Crete* (New York: Harper Collins, 1999) The much-touted Mediterranean diet, including recipes and complete menus.

Elizabeth Somer, *Nutrition For Women: The Complete Guide* (New York: Owl Books, 1995) A comprehensive guide for women on how to make changes and maintain good health. Includes shopping guides and other valuable information.

Andrew Weil, M.D., *Eating Well For Optimum Health* (New York: Alfred Knopf, 2000) Informative facts on nutrition, and healthful eating to improve well being, and reduce the risk of disease.

Rebecca Wood, *The New Whole Foods Encyclopedia* (New York: Penguin Books, 1999) Alphabetized reference book that runs the gamut from the preparation, selection and storage for over 1,000 fruits, vegetables, grains and herbs to healing techniques that incorporate Ayurveda, western nutrition and traditional Chinese medicine.

www.cavemandiet.com is dedicated to replacing American's typical diet of processed foods and cultivated grains, with lean meats, fish, fresh fruits and vegetables, nuts, berries and seeds. The site also provides an historical background on a variety of ancient diets. Check it out.

www.eatright.org is a site of the American Dietetic Association. Registered dietitians will answer consumer questions via e-mail.

www.epicurious.com is a fun-site for people who love to eat, and want to become more knowledgeable about food. Something for everyone whether they just like to eat or consider themselves a gourmet.

www.heartinfo.com describes how to give obesity and heart disease a one, two punch. Check out the Nutrition Guide for ways to improve over-all health.

www.mayohealth.org the Mayo Clinic's Nutrition Center provides the services of a dietician to transform your favorite recipes to more healthful versions. Learn more about problem foods, and the latest information on healthful choices. Check out the virtual cookbook.

www.mealsforyou.com is recipe heaven. Do you have an ingredient but no recipe to use it in? This site will provide the recipe along with preparation instructions and nutritional information.

www.nal.usda.gov/fnic/ is the U.S. Department of Agriculture Food and Nutrition Information Center. The site has volumes of information on food choices, nutrition, dietary guidelines, reports and studies, and more. It's very informative.

www.northcoast.com/~alden/cookhome.html is the "The Cooks Thesaurus". Need an alternative ingredient for a recipe—this site has lots of low fat, low calorie, inexpensive, and hard-to-find suggestions to assist in meal preparation.

www.soyfoods.com is all about soy products from tofu to tempeh—how to find, prepare, and incorporate soy into meals. Provides lots of additional information, including research results and nutritional benefits.

www.vegsource.com will help individuals who may be thinking about becoming vegetarians, or simply want to make some dietary changes. This site provides the information you need, including answers from the experts.

www.vrg.org includes recipes, nutrition information, where to find vegetarian food in your travels, a game to test your knowledge of vegetarianism and more.

Appendix C

Exercise Resources

Books and Websites

Karen Aneles and the editor's of Fitness Magazine, *The Complete Book of Fitness: Mind, Body, Spirit* (New York: Three Rivers Press, 1999) A compendium for everyone on strength and cardiovascular training, nutrition and other methods for promoting wellness.

Beryl Bender Birch, *Power Yoga,* (New York: Macmillan Publishing Company, 1995) This form of yoga takes all the major muscle groups through a complete workout. Best done by individuals who are well on the way to becoming, or already are, physically fit.

Elise Browning Miller and Carol Blackman, *Easy Yoga, Anytime, Anywhere* (St. Paul, MN: Llewellyn Publications, 1999) Offers simple step-by-step methods to increase endurance, strength, and flexibility, plus proper breathing techniques, which combine to make you feel years younger.

Annette Cain, *Get In Shape: The Lazy Way,* (New York: MacMillan General Reference, 1999) Learn some simple and engaging methods for body toning and shaping.

Alice Christensen, *The American Yoga Association's Easy Does It Yoga,* (New York: Fireside, 1999) A way to fitness for those who are challenged by age, illness, injury or inactivity.

Michael Gerrish, *When Working Out Isn't Working Out: A Mind/Body Guide to Conquering Unidentified Fitness Obstacles,* (New York: St.

Martin's Griffin, 1999) If you're having trouble meeting your exercise goals, help has arrived. The author guides the reader past UFO's (Unidentified Fitness Obstacles).

Julie T. Lusk, *Desktop Yoga*, (New York: A Perigee Book, 1998) Bring this book to work and rejuvenate your body and mind within only minutes, with exercises you can do at your desk.

Mira Mehta, *How to Use Yoga*, (Berkeley, CA:Rodmell Press, 1998) An easy to follow yoga program meant to reduce stress and improve health and overall well-being. Beautiful color photos illustrate the postures. This book is suitable for everyone from beginners to experts.

Casey Meyers, *Walking: A Complete Guide to a Complete Exercise*, (New York: Random House, 1992) A concise tome that encompasses the principles, benefits and requirements of walking.

Suzanne Schlosberg, *The Ultimate Workout Log* (New York: Houghton Mifflin Company, 1998) It's a log, it's a guide—and if you're prepared to stick with a regular exercise routine this book will support your efforts and keep track of how far you've come.

Porter Shimer, *Too Busy To Exercise* (Pownal, VT: Storey Publishing, 1996) A no excuses accepted book that explains how to fit exercise into a daily schedule.

Kathy Smith (audio tape) *Kathy Smith's Walking Easy*, (Time Warner Audio Books) one of several excellent audio tapes from KM that will keep you walking.

Joyce Vedral, *12-Minute Total Body Workout*, (Fawcett Books, New York, 1995) No need for expensive equipment when you follow this workout.

You can e-mail the author at *jvbody@aol.com* for tips and answers to questions you may have.

Gary Yanker, *Exercise RX: A Lifetime Prescription for Reducing Medical Risks and Sport Injuries* (New York: Kodansha America, Inc., 1999) A how-to book and medical reference guide that will help individuals incorporate exercise into their daily life.

http://www2.gdi.net/~mjm/resource.html (Yoga Resources) site for supplementing yoga classes or practice—includes information on books, videos and postures (asanas).

www.acefitness.org offers the latest information on health facts and trends, fitness, sporting equipment and workout apparel.

www.asimba.com is staffed with health experts who create customized workouts and nutrition plans free of charge. It has lots of how-to information, especially ways to say on track.

www.50plus.org is dedicated to fitness for individual's 50 and over, but those under 50 are welcome too. Need help in getting started with an exercise program then check out the newsletter "Taking the First Step". The bi-monthly publication offers professional answers to health and fitness questions. Membership fee.

www.fitnesszone.com provides a personalized fitness profile plus nutrition and exercise plans. Find a local gym and utilize the classified section to buy or sell equipment.

www.healthwalk.com offers information on Walkers Club of America. For those who are interested in walking—whether fitness walking or power walking—join up with fellow walkers to stay motivated.

http://members.aol.com/rayzwocker/worldclass/homepage.htm is Dave's World Class Racewalking site. Provides a variety of information on the subject.

www.phys.com is packed with information on fitness, exercise, nutrition, weight loss, diet, and more. Check out the workout slide shows.

www.shapeup.org is Shape Up America's web site offering plenty of information on getting in shape and staying that way, from evaluating your body's fitness to ways to improve it.

www.thrive.net/shape/women.fit.html focuses on getting fit and staying fit with lots of helpful tips and programs.

www.women.com/fitness focuses on weight training, weight loss and walking. Sign on to the message boards to exchange questions and ideas with other women.

Appendix D

Stress Management Resources

Books and Websites

Robert Anthony, *50 Ideas That Can Change Your Life* (New York: Berkley, 1982) Timeless suggestions for staying on track and improving your life

Mark Bricklin & Linda Konner, *Your Perfect Weight* (Emmaus, PA: Rodale Press, 1995) An in-your-face recipe for incorporating diet, exercise and stress management into everyday life, and lots of day-by-day techniques that promote success.

Deepak Chopra, M.D., *Perfect Health: The Complete Mind/Body Guide* (New York: Harmony Books, 1991) If you want to learn how to achieve a natural balance via Ayrveda medicine, based on the mind/body connection, check it out.

Harold H. Bloomfield, M.D., *Healing Anxiety Naturally* (New York: Harper Collins, 1999), Learn how to use herbal medicine to relieve stress, anxiety and insomnia.

Peter G. Hanson, M.D., *The Joy of Stress: How To Make Stress Work For You* (Kansas City, KS Andrews & McMeel, 1985) Good advice on how to take stress and turn it around so that it becomes an effective tool for improving your life.

Jon Kabat-Zinn, *Full Catastrophe Living: Using the Wisdom of Your Body and Mind to Face Stress, Pain and Illness* (New York: Dell Publishing, 1991) Details how to use mindfulness to cope with illness and daily tensions.

Ada P. Kahn, *Stress A-Z: A Sourcebook For Facing Everyday Challenges,* (New York: Facts On File, Inc) Explains the multiple factors that promote stress and provides resources to help get back on tract.

Vernon M. Sylvert, M.D., *The Formula: Who Gets Sick, Who Get Well, Who is Happy, Who is Unhappy and Why,* (Fairfield, IA: Sunstar Publishing Ltd, 1999) Sustain a happy healthy and spiritually productive life through integration of spiritual traditions and western healing.

Stephanie Tourles, *50 Simple Ways to Pamper Yourself,* (Pownal, VT: Storey Books, 1999) Tips for nourishing and rejuvenating your body and mind.

www.meditatenow.com/stress.htm suggests various stress reduction methods, and has links to meditations.

www.mediconsult.com/mc/mcsite.nsf/conditionnav/stress-sectionintroduction provides stress and anxiety information—from causes to management.

www.stresstips.com offers all sorts of support for managing a variety of stresses.

www.suite101.com/welcome.cfm/stress_management furnishes helpful ways to reduce stress, with links to related topics.

www.pp.okstate.edu/ehs/links/stress.htm provides a variety of articles, information and resources for stress management.

Index

References

[1] Ries LAG, Kosary CL, et al (eds). *SEER Cancer Statistics Review 1973-1995*. National Cancer Institute. Bethesda, MD. 1998

[2] "Cancer Facts and Figures for African American 1998-1999, *American Cancer Society,* 1998

[3] Garfinkel, L., et al. "Changing trends: An overview of breast cancer incidence and mortality". *Cancer. 1994; 74: 222-227.*

[4] Ries LAG, Kosary CL, et al. *SEER Cancer Statistics Review, 1973-1994: Tables and Graphs.* Bethesda, MD: National Cancer Institute; 1997.

[5] "Cancer Facts and Figures for African Americans 1998-1999", *American Cancer Society*, 1998

[6] "Cancer Facts and Figures, 2001", *American Cancer Society*, 2001

[7] Ries LAG, Kosary CL, et al. *SEER Cancer Statistics Review, 1973-1994: Tables and Graphs.* Bethesda, MD: National Cancer Institute; 1997.

[8] "Breast Cancer in Black Women." *Annals of Internal Medicine*, May 15, 1996; 124(10): 875-905

[9] Rochefordiere, et al. 1993. "Age as prognostic factor in pre-menopausal breast cancer." *Lancet,* 341: 1039-1043

10 Hughes and Jones. "Intake of dietary fiber and the age of menarche." *Annals of Human Biology*, 1985: 325-332

11 Love, Susan Dr. *Dr. Susan Love's Breast Book.* Addison Wesley Publishing Company, 1995

12 Struewing, Jeffery P., Patricia Hartge, et al. "The Risk of Cancer Associated with Specific Mutations of BRCA1 and BRCA2 Among Ashkenazi Jews." NEJM: May 15, 1997, 336, 20: 1401-1408

13 Ambrose, C.B., et al. 1995. "N-acetyltransferase (NAT), cigarette smoking, and breast cancer risk." *Proc Am Assoc Cancer Res*; 36: 283 (abstract)

14 "Smoking and Tobacco Control", Monograph 4. pp. v and vii. *DHHS*, 1993; NIH Pub. No. 93-360

15 Longnecker, M.P. 1994. "Alcoholic beverage consumption in relation to risk of breast cancer: meta-analysis and renew." *Cancer Causes Control* 5: 23-32

16 Bowlin, Steven J. Dr., et al. "Breast cancer risk and alcohol consumption: results from a large case-control study". *International Journal of Epidemiology* 1997;26:915-923

17 "Alcohol may pose problems for women on estrogen." *Tufts University Health & Nutrition Letter*. Feb 1997,12: 1-2

18 Tannenbaum, A. "Nutrition and Cancer." *Physiopathy of Cancer*, 2nd ed., ed. F. Homberger. New York: Hoeber-Harper, 517-62

[19] Ballard-Barbesh, et al. 1990. "Body fat distribution and breast cancer in the Framingham study." *Journal National Cancer Institute* 82: 286-290

[20] Monson, Richard R. ed. "Cancer Causes & Control. An International Journal of Studies of Cancer in Human Populations", *Harvard Report on Cancer Prevention*, Nov 1996; 7(1):S11-13

[21] Huang Z, et al. "Dual effects of weight and weight gain on breast cancer risk". *JAMA* 1997 Nov5;278 (17): 1407-1411

[22] Miller, A.B. et al. 1989. "Mortality from breast cancer after irradiation during fluoroscopic examinations in patients being treated for tuberculosis." *New England Journal of Medicine*; 321: 1285-89

[23] Hancock, S.L. et al. 1993. "Breast cancer after treatment of Hodgkin's disease." *Journal of the National Cancer Institute*; 85: 25-31

[24] Wolff, M., Toniolo, G. et al. "Blood levels of organochorine residues and risk of breast cancer." *Journal of the National Cancer Institute*, 1993; 85: 648-52

[25] Dewailly M.S., Dodin S. et al. "High organochlorine body burden in women with estrogen receptor-positive breast cancer." *J. Natl Cancer Inst 1994, 86(3):232-234*

[26] Aronson K.J., Miller A.B. et al. "Breast adipose tissue concentrations of polychlorinated biphenyls and other organochlorines and breast cancer risk." *Cancer Epidemiol Biomarkers Prev* 2000 Jan;9(1):55-63

[27] Hunter, D.J., Hankinson, S.E., Laden, F., et al. "Plasma organocholorine levels and the risk of breast cancer." *New England Journal of Medicine*, 1997:337(18);1253-1258

28 Krieger N, Wolff M.S. et al. "Breast cancer and serum organochlorines: a prospective study among white, black, and Asian women." *J Natl Cancer Inst* 1994 Apr 20; 86(8): 589-99

29 Kang, K.S., Wilson, M.R. et al. "Inhibition of gap junctional intercellular communication in normal human breast epithelial cells after treatment with pesticides, PCBs and PBBs, alone or in mixtures." *Environmental Health Perspectives* 1996 104(2):192-200

30 Decensi A, Bonanni B, et al. "Biologic activity of tamoxifen at low doses in healthy women". *J Natl Cancer Inst* 1998 Oct 7;90(19):1461-7

31 Gail MH, Costantino JP, et al. "Weighing the risks and benefits of tamoxifen treatment for preventing breast cancer." *J Natl Cancer Inst* 1999 Nov 3;91(21):1829-46

32 Cummings, SR, et al. "The effect of raloxifene on risk of breast cancer in postmenopausal women: results from the MORE randomized trial." *JAMA 1999* June 16;281(23):2189-97

33 Putnam, Judith Jones and Jane E. Allshouse. "Food Consumption, Prices and Expenditures 1970-97." Food and Rural Economics Division, Economic Research Service, U.S. Dept. of Agriculture, Statistical Bulletin No. 965.

34 Holmes, Michelle Dr. et al. "Association of dietary intake of fat and fatty acids with risk of breast cancer." *JAMA* 1999 March 10:281(10):914-20

35 *Archives of Internal Medicine* 1998; 158:1181-1187

[36] 1993. *Journal National Cancer Institute* 85: 1819

[37] Deschner EE, et al. "The effect of dietary omega-3 fatty acids (fish oil) on azoxymethanol-induced focal areas of dysplasia and colon tumor incidence." *Cancer* 1990;66:2350-6.

[38] Gabor H, et al. "Effect of dietary fat and monoclonal antibody therapy on the growth of human mammary adenocarcinoma MX-1 grafted in athymic mice". *Cancer Lett* 1990;52:173-8.

[39] Hubbard NE, et al. "Alteration of murine mammary tumorigenesis by dietary enrichment with n-3fatty acids in fish oil". Cancer Lett 1998: Feb 13;124(1):1-7

[40] Kaizer L. et al. "Fish consumption and breast cancer risk: an ecological study". *Nutrition and Cancer* 1989;12:61-68.

[41] Rose, DP. "Dietary fatty acids and prevention of hormone-responsive cancer." *Proc Soc Exp Biol Med,* 1997 Nov;216(2):224-33

[42] Kohlmeier, Lenore Dr. et al. "Adipose tissue trans fatty acids and breast cancer in the European Community Multicenter Study on antioxidants, myocardial infarction, and breast cancer." *Cancer Epidemiology Biomarkers Prev* 1997 Sep;6(9):705-710

[43] Hu, FB, et al. "Dietary Fat intake and the risk of coronary heart disease in women." *N Engl J Med* 1997 Nov 20;337:1491-1499

[44] Kelly SM, et al. "A 3-month, double-blind, controlled trial of feeding with sucrose polyester in human volunteers." *Br J Nutr* 1998 Jul;80(1):41-9

45 Food Surveys Research Group. Pyramid servings data: results for USDA's 1995 and 1996 Continuing Survey of Food Intakes by Individuals. Riverdale, MD: *USDA Agricultural Research Service*, 1997

46 Burton-Freeman, B. "Dietary fiber and energy regulation." *Journal of Nutrition*, Feb 2000; 130(2S Supl):272S-275S

47 Rose DP, et al. "Effects of diet supplementation with wheat bran on serum estrogen levels in the follicular and luteal phases of the menstrual cycle". *Nutrition* 1997 Jun;13(6):535-9

48 Swanson, CA, et al. "Alcohol consumption and breast cancer risk among women under age 45 years." *Epidemiology,* 1997 May; 8(3):231-7

49 Bland JS. "Phytonutrition, phytotherapy, and phytopharmacology." *Altern Ther Health Med* 1996 Nov;2(6):73-6

50 "Exercise reduces cancer." *Cancer Researcher Weekly*, October 3, 1994: 1

51 Thune, Inger, M.D., et al. "Physical Activity and the Risk of Breast Cancer." *The New England Journal of Medicine 336*(18):1269-1312, May 1, 1997.

52 "Biomarkers and prevention." *Cancer Epidemiology*, March 1996

53 *Journal National Cancer Institute 1996 88:650*

54 Hirose K, et.al. "Effect of body size on breast-cancer risk among Japanese women". *Int J Cancer* 1999 Jan 29;80(3):349-55

55 Blair, et al. 1989. "Physical fitness, an all cause mortality." *JAMA* 262:2395-2401

56 "Heart disease and women: Be physically active." *National Institutes of Health*, August 1995

57 Dalsky GP. "The role of exercise in the prevention of osteoporosis". *Compr Ther* 1989 Sep;15(9):30-7

58 Forbes, GB. "The adult decline in lean body mass". *Human Biology* 1976: 48, 161-73

59 "Can yoga make you fit?" *The University of California, Berkeley Wellness Letter*. May 1997, 6

60 Chen, C.C., et al. "Adverse life events and breast cancer: case-control study." *British Medical Journal* 1995: 152-155

61 Seyle H. *Stress in Health and Disease*. London, UK: Buttersworth, 1976

62 Astin, JA. "Stress reduction through mindfulness meditation. Effects on psychological symptomatology, sense of control, and spiritual experiences." *Psychother Psychosom*, 1997, 66:2, 97-106

Printed in the United States
137222LV00002B/1/A

9 780595 158317